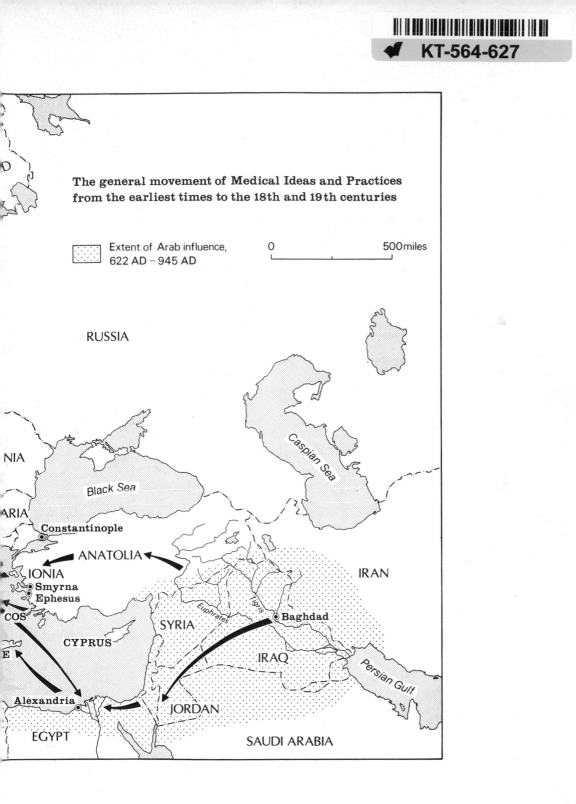

The general movement of Medical Ideas and Practices
from the earliest times to the 18th and 19th centuries

Extent of Arab influence,
622 AD – 945 AD

0   500 miles

RUSSIA

Caspian Sea

Black Sea

NIA

ARIA

Constantinople

ANATOLIA

IRAN

IONIA

Smyrna

Ephesus

COS

Euphrates

Tigris

Baghdad

SYRIA

CYPRUS

IRAQ

Persian Gulf

Alexandria

JORDAN

EGYPT

SAUDI ARABIA

An Outline History of Medicine

Philip Rhodes, MA, MB, BChir(Cantab), FRCS, FRCOG, FRACMA

Professor of Postgraduate Medical Education, University of Southampton, and Dean of Graduate Medicine, Wessex Region of the National Health Service
Formerly Postgraduate Dean of Medicine, University of Newcastle upon Tyne; Dean of the Faculty of Medicine, University of Adelaide, South Australia; Dean of St. Thomas's Hospital Medical School, London

Butterworths
London Boston Durban Singapore Sydney Toronto Wellington

First published, 1985

© Philip Rhodes, 1985

British Library Cataloguing in Publication Data

Rhodes, Philip
  An outline history of medicine.
  1. Medicine——History
  I. Title
  610′.9   R131

  ISBN 0-407-00410-6
  ISBN 0-407 00343-6 Pbk

Library of Congress Cataloging in Publication Data

Rhodes, Philip.
  An outline history of medicine.

  Bibliography: p.
  Includes indexes.
  1. Medicine——History——Outlines, syllabi, etc.
2. Science——History——Outlines, syllabi, etc. I. Title.
[DNLM: 1. History of Medicine. WZ 40 R4770]
R131.R47 1985 610′.9   84-23137
ISBN 0-407-00410-6
ISBN 0-407-00343-6 (pbk.)

Typeset by Phoenix Photosetting, Chatham
Printed in Great Britain at the University Press, Cambridge

Preface

This is not meant to be a textbook of the history of medicine in the usual tradition. There are many excellent major works on the subject, some of which are mentioned in the bibliography. There are histories of the various subjects of medicine, biology and science too, along with hundreds of biographies of the famous. Some deal with specific periods of medicine, or that of various cultures and countries. The choice is overwhelming for the general interested reader. This can mean that he or she does not even begin. It is the intention of this book that readers should give the subject a try. The reasons for offering such temptation are that the history of medicine is fascinating in its own right; it gives perspective to modern medicine and where it is heading; it gives insight into what may be lasting and what ephemeral; and it sheds light on some of the philosophical and ethical problems of today, which are an increasing concern of the medical profession, other health care workers and society at large.

It is because of these concerns that the book constantly tries to put medicine in its scientific and social contexts. Medicine cannot be isolated from its life and times. It springs from and adds to its intellectual environment. There is constant interaction between them, often unperceived on either side. In some senses therefore this is a cultural history, and it does not attempt to list every major contributor to medicine, nor every advance that has been made. Instead it tries to develop a history of ideas in medicine—the ways in which they have been derived and from which intellectual places—and how they have been translated into action by a few outstanding people who especially interpret the spirit of their ages, making that more apparent and obvious to their contemporaries as well as to their successors and inheritors. Often, of course, it is only in retrospect that the significance of a person's life, work, observations and experiments is more clearly recognized. Significance depends on the standpoints, predilections and presuppositions of those who observe the phenomena. Those of this author will readily become evident for any reader.

So this is an introduction to an immense subject, meant to be read in a short time and give an outline sketch with some facts and interpretation in a general historical perspective as perceived by the writer. This has been developed over more than 30 years by diffuse and dilettante reading, as any professional will rapidly realize. Yet there has been some direction in that over this period a chronology has been compiled in which any detail of history, science, philosophy, biology, medicine and literature to which some date can be given has been entered under the appropriate year, since AD 1500. This at least has given the opportunity to see some broad general sweeps in the history of ideas and to some extent relate medicine to them. It is this that forms the basis of what is written here.

Because of this somewhat novel approach, without an overload of fact and an emphasis on principles, it is hoped that there will be an attraction for medical students and doctors, as well as science students and the general reader. The student and doctor of today is so overwhelmed with facts that there is little time in which to raise the eyes to the horizons and enjoy the view by reference to the past, and possibly to the future.

If what is presented here may help a few to do this, then I shall be well content. It will not matter if those few disagree with all or some of what is written. They will for a while have stopped, looked and listened and above all considered something of the place of medicine within the scheme of things. That is what I hope to provoke them to do. It is the function of the teacher and author to bring this about. His task is not simply to disgorge facts to be memorized but to ask that those who read or listen shall consider, weigh and take delight in thinking about what goes on around them, making appropriate estimates and assessments of significance. Thus will attitudes and value judgements be made. On these all else depends in action. Without historical perspective they will lack a more sure base than they ought to have.

P.R.
Southampton and Brockenhurst

Acknowledgements

An author always needs help, both explicit and implicit. My secretary, Mary Bartlett, has patiently typed and retyped the manuscript and has combed the libraries for sources. Peter Richardson, the editor for Butterworths, has retained enthusiasm for the project and has maintained my morale, as well as taking on many of the chores inseparable from book production. Mr William Schupback at the Wellcome Institute Library, London, has kindly provided almost all the illustrations. My wife has been forebearing and supportive. Above all I am grateful to innumerable teachers and authors who have shaped my education even though they might not be very satisfied with it, nor be conscious of their influence. Nor can I always know who they were and are.

Contents

Introduction

The pattern of this book is essentially chronological, tracing the development of medicine from guesswork about the actions of prehistoric Man through the centuries to some aspects of the present day. The intellectual and cultural centres of the world have moved over time from place to place. Not only have they dominated socially, economically, politically and militarily, they have also carried the arts, sciences, humanities and philosophies with them, whether or not they are now deemed to have progressed or regressed in these various endeavours. It is of importance to recognize that progress in medicine, as we visualize it, rarely, if ever, occurs in isolation. It follows in the wake of and is part of general progress. Civilizations seem to advance on many fronts at once. They develop an intellectual climate which feeds and sustains, and is exemplified in, several fields, with ideas crossing and re-crossing boundaries between subjects, which for clarity of thought about them we separate. This is because our own highly specialized society has had to separate them. In earlier times all knowledge was part of a conglomerate which one polymath might be able to master in a way no longer open to anyone now. These omnicompetents, often thought of as philosophers, moved easily from speculation to practicality, from art to science and from peace to war. They were, by our standards, relatively unconfined and free to move over the range of human existence as then known. This shows one of the historically persistent patterns in the move from generalization to specialization over long periods of time.

Despite the several civilizations that have come and gone in many parts of the world, this book inevitably concentrates on medicine in the western part of it, mainly because that is where the lead is now, and also because that is the perspective of the writer. So from primitive Man the move is to the first civilization of the Fertile Crescent of Mesopotamia, bounded by the valleys of the rivers Tigris and Euphrates, and ancient Egypt. There is comparatively little to say of this period in medicine, in four or five thousand years before Christ.

The first awakening of medicine, for present purposes, belongs to the time of classical Greece, when medicine was based essentially on the teachings of Hippocrates and his followers. This might be said to extend roughly from his birth c.460 BC to the decline of Greece and the dominance of Rome in the few centuries around the dawn of the Christian era. At this time the intellectual centre for medicine moved from Athens to Alexandria and then on to Rome. However, it is not to be thought that the theories and practice of medicine important to us were in any way confined to these cities. Their influence and culture spread far and wide through the known world, and especially along the shores of the Mediterranean.

With the decline of Rome came the Middle Ages, based in feudalism and dominated by the church which had a virtual monopoly of knowledge and learning. As regards medicine the clergy did little in this period, for it was the age of Scholasticism concerned with religious dogma and interpretation. But in the early part of the period c.600–700 came the rise of Islam, and Arabic physicians preserved and advanced the earlier Greek medicine, so that its ideas and methods were extant again along the northern and southern shores of the Mediterranean as far as Spain and Morocco from the base in the Middle East.

For reasons to be explored later the yoke of Scholasticism on medicine began to be thrown off with the Renaissance around the fifteenth century. This was essentially based in northern Italy, and saw the beginnings of sound observational anatomy. The real scientific era had then begun. The intellectual spirit of the Renaissance spread throughout Europe and especially northwards to Paris, Holland and England, as well as into Switzerland and Germany and the Scandinavian countries. And early in the seventeenth century Harvey published his work on the circulation of the blood and the motion of the heart. This was the result of observation, inference and most significantly experiment, so that another dimension was added to medical advance. Later in the seventeenth century Newton revolutionized the whole way of looking at the physical world, with profound consequences for natural science, including medicine.

The eighteenth century brought further advances, especially in midwifery with the advent of the obstetric forceps, and the scientific approach of John Hunter to surgery. Almost unconsciously the methods of observation, careful recording, inference, hypothesis and experiment had been learned from the pioneers and were being applied in a variety of directions and subjects. Chemistry had begun to progress as a result of the researches of Boyle, Hooke, Priestley and many others.

The nineteenth century was dominated by Charles Darwin, who changed the way of looking at the living world, just as Newton had done for the physical world. It is impossible to estimate just how much these two have brought about in the later working out of their ideas, experiments and speculations. But the later nineteenth century saw the beginnings of bacteriology and of cellular pathology, and by the turn of the century psychiatry had started, largely as a result of the work of Freud and many others.

The twentieth century has been the age of specialization as scientific knowledge and its applications have burgeoned. About the middle of the century came the therapeutic explosion based on increasingly rational pharmacy and the application of physics and chemistry and other sciences and technologies in the service of medicine.

The key words in this tracing of the story of medicine might then be:

  Prehistoric.
  Ancient civilization (Fertile Crescent).
  Greece (Hippocrates).
  Alexandria.
  Rome (Galen).
  Arabia.
  Middle Ages.

Renaissance (anatomy, observation).
Harvey (experiment).
Newton (physics).
Chemistry.
Darwin (biology).
Specialization.

These are to be thought of as peaks epitomizing certain epochs of thought and action in the development of medicine. These epochs are not to be demarcated rigidly from one another, and they are not to be confined within decades or even centuries. The history of thought is that of a slow shading off of one form into that of another, almost imperceptibly. Ideas and actions, consonant with their times, arise and diffuse, and thereafter may flourish, stagnate, die or lie torpidly until awakened once more when the time is ripe.

The general course of the history of medicine is from massive speculation—without allowing it to be much influenced by fact, as observed or derived from experiment—to narrower and narrower smaller hypotheses, potentially testable by observation and experiment. There is a move too from supernatural to natural explanations of phenomena; and it all takes a very long time, with the old clinging to the new, impeding its progress and having to be discarded as time passes, so that novel and fruitful ways of looking at events may emerge and be tested. In short, medicine is one aspect of the development of scientific method being applied in one of the most difficult areas of nature. For medicine has little justification except as a practice. It must be a practical art, or science, or both (whichever word you prefer).

In slightly more specific terms the mind concerned with medicine first speculates about a problem, then tries to solve it empirically with the tools available at the time. In the earliest times these tools could only be some modifications of the diet, bathing, rest and sleep, with perhaps some potions of doubtful value. In investigations too, as far as these were undertaken, there was little at hand that could be used. But then there may come technological advances, perhaps outside medicine, which may be applicable within it. An hypothesis can be tested and may have to be modified by the facts disclosed by the new technique, and then that in its turn may have to be modified. There is constant interplay between hypothesis and technology. It is obvious enough that cellular biology and pathology were not possible until the microscope had been invented, and that the further development of electron microscopy had to wait on the appropriate moves in electronics. The whole gamut of investigational and many therapeutic techniques, so prominent a feature of modern medicine, have come from technological advances, not normally thought of as belonging within the usual definitions of medicine. And whole specialties have grown out of some of these technques.

Sometimes progress may occur because of a change in social attitudes. Such was needed before anatomy could be undertaken, when the human body was no longer seen as totally sacred. And it is social changes that have made termination of pregnancy more acceptable.

It is hoped that the reader will keep these various generalities in mind as he comes across apparently specific advances attributed to one person. They do not happen by one person's agency alone, but arise from the climate of opinion and knowledge of the times, both in general and within the subject concerned. The act of creation lies in seeing in a new way what is to everyone's hand, and in juxtaposing and reconciling facts and hypotheses, whose relevance to each other had not before been realized. This is the marvellous intellectual achievement that we honour. We receive and use gifts from the past of which we are often unaware. Many of them now form the basis of today's theory and practice of medicine. They were hardly won in their time, though now they are rightly taken for granted, and used because they are established. And this too is a use of history, for it shows that the miracles and breakthroughs of today will in their turn become the commonplace of tomorrow, and that we are no less prone to error than our ancestors were, and which only our progeny will recognize.

Chapter 1

The beginnings

The mind of primitive Man and much of his technology are now unfathomable. A certain amount of knowledge of the functioning of primitive tribes can be gleaned from researches in social anthropology. There are usually what we might categorize as priests, law-givers and medicine-men. The functions of magic, religion, interpretation of customs, of healing and propitiation might all be combined in one man, and there is no easy separation of these various activities. The medicine-man may be seen as a magician in touch with supernatural powers, who if influenced by appropriate spells, incantations and potions might be expected to do his bidding. One has to try to understand the reasons for such beliefs and imagine what it must be like to be with a few others of your tribe in a hostile environment.

The world must appear awe inspiring. There are the winds, the rain, storms, night, day, stars, sun, moon, seasons, birth, life, disease and death, all to be explained. And there is the unremitting struggle for food, warmth and shelter. Man does seek explanations, for that is the basis of being a social, communicating animal. When something happens, particularly if it is catastrophic, there has to be a theory as to why. When there is total ignorance of the relationships of natural phenomena, then the supernatural is invoked. There are gods, demons and spirits which control everything, sometimes benignly and sometimes with malign intent, sometimes to help and sometimes to punish. These powers may be insubstantial or they may inhabit rocks, stones, places or take on human, animal or plant shape. They are everywhere: They move the heavens, they determine whether crops and herds shall flourish or fail, they ride the storms and the waters, and they control human individual destiny. Above all they are capricious and their actions are unpredictable. They then have to be calmed and appeased by propitiation and sacrifice. In the daily grip of such powers individual helplessness has to be minimized by turning to experts. These are the priest and the medicine-man, often combined in one person.

The parallels with today are obvious. So often when we are in trouble we turn to the doctor, the priest or the lawyer. Their functions are needed for the understanding and control of the natural, the supernatural and the relationships between members of society. It was not, however, until mediaeval times, when universities were founded, that the separation of functions was firmly established in the faculties of medicine, law and theology, with theology as the senior discipline. And in those times and earlier, medicine included much of what we would designate as natural science. Doctors were not only medical practitioners, they were men of science too, and often much else besides in the culture of their times.

Primitive medicine-men understood the behaviour of the supernatural and the natural, and how they affected their patients. They must have been able to cope with many varieties of injury. Broken bones obviously need straightening and to be held still by splinting and bandaging for the relief of pain. In the 1970s in Australia an Aborigine woman was partially buried in sand to immobilize her broken thigh. It is interesting too that there are many examples of healed fractures in apes, such as gorillas, chimpanzees, orang-utans and gibbons, and in monkeys and other animals. There is therefore no reason to suppose that men and women did not recover from fractured limbs in the distant past, just as dinosaurs are known to have done. And there is evidence too of recovery of ancient man from skull fractures of various kinds.

Since animal skins were sewn together for clothing it is highly likely too that human skin lacerations were sutured after a fashion. Dressings for wounds might very well have been smeared with various concoctions, including fats, and resins, and possibly honey, which is still on trial occasionally today. For the pain of injury there was often alcohol to be taken in one of its various forms, for fermentation of substances of many different kinds is virtually ubiquitious. There were almost certainly various herbs, roots, leaves and parts of animals used for similar purposes. The coca shrub, for instance, is widely growing in the southern hemisphere. From its leaves cocaine is extracted, and some of its properties were apparent to many tribes, the best known being the Peruvian Indians. There are probably many other such plants with properties still not known to modern pharmacology for alleviation and cure of illness.

Warmth or cold applied locally or generally to the sick and injured are obvious enough too; that is using the technology that is immediately available. Cooling the fevered brow or applying heat to an abdomen afflicted with gastroenteritis must have been discovered very early. It is obvious too that the sick feel the need for different diets than those eaten when they are well, and this has always been part of nursing care, together with the tenderness and compassion inseparable from the proper conduct of that profession.

Injury and the butchery of killed animals must have led to rudimentary understanding of anatomy. The viscera—brain, heart, lungs, liver, guts, muscles and bones—must all have been recognizable, though without systematization of that crude knowledge, nor recognition of pathological conditions. But trephining of the skull is known to have been practised several thousand years BC (*Figure 1.1*), and the skulls subjected to this have been shown to have both healed and healing edges of the holes deliberately made in the skull dome. It is believed that this was probably done to allow the egress of evil spirits, perhaps thought to be causing strange behaviour or constant headaches. This is of interest since it suggests that it was understood that mental phenomena belonged to the brain, and it suggests an empirical knowledge of anatomy so that the saw cuts could be made in places away from blood vessels of the scalp and the great sinuses of the brain.

For other demonic possessions such as might afflict the organs of the chest, abdomen or spine there was probably no surgery, except the opening of abscesses, but rather the use of some potions to be taken by mouth, as a sort of witches' brew, made up by the medicine-man. But in addition there was belief that the body could only be rid of evil spirits by various forms of magic, much of which was kept secret or remained in a family, being handed down from father to son.

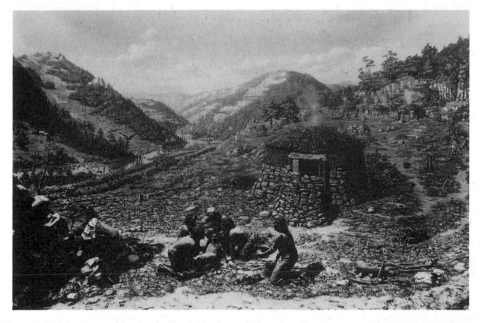

Figure 1.1 Diorama: trephination in Neolithic times. (Reproduced by courtesy of the Wellcome Institute Library, London)

Yet in surgery there is evidence that caesarean section was performed in India a few thousand years BC. It may be that this was done after the death of a pregnant mother, rather than on the living, though this is not certain. It is just possible that if the abdominal section was performed at the instant of death a living child might result, as occasionally happens today.

Of course much of this has to be speculation, but there is perhaps enough evidence from the anthropological sciences to show that it is not entirely fanciful and has some plausibility. Also, the fossil record of Man shows that he suffered from injury, congenital abnormalities (e.g. dwarfism), scurvy, bone tumours (benign and malignant), inflammations, arthritis, dental diseases, tuberculosis and leprosy. All these can make imprints on the skeletal tissues. So there has never been a golden age when Man was free of disease, nor has there been for other animals investigated palaeontologically (*Figure 1.2*). Disease and injury are inseparable from living.

This primitive basis of medicine is still with us consisting of care and compassion for the sick and injured, with nursing, the use of available drugs and surgery, varying the diet, and appealing to the supernatural when the man-made efforts fail. This still happens with patients even when they and their scientific doctors may not believe in anything supernatural themselves. It is a phase in the psychological processes of dying in most patients. Doctors and scientists appeal for further research; two words that complete a large number of scientific papers, when the authors cannot proceed further and are stumped. Is this an appeal to the god of science, so perpetuating a very ancient tradition?

With recorded history of a kind beginning in Mesopotamia there seem to have been a few physicians, since their seals have been discovered. But it was later in

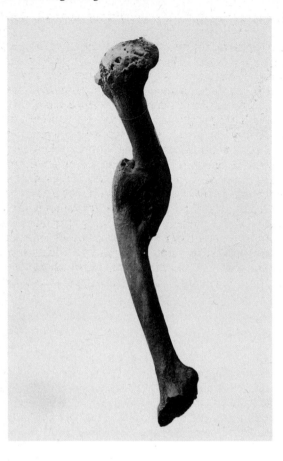

Figure 1.2 Egyptian thigh bone with badly healed fracture. (Berlin Museum) (Reproduced by courtesy of the Wellcome Institute Library, London)

Babylon about 1900 BC that King Hammurabi drew up a Code of Laws, some of which concerned medicine, laying down the payments to be made to a doctor who was successful in the treatment of a patient, either master or slave, in such as the opening of an abscess or the preservation of sight. But also it laid down penalties for failure of treatment, extending from payment for injury to having his hand cut off!

From that time the next documentary evidence comes from the Ebers Papyrus, named after its discoverer and found in a tomb of Thebes on the Nile, near Luxor. The papyrus is a medical text, accurately dated as 1550 BC. It is full of spells and incantations and strange remedies for a variety of diseases, including crocodile bite. The remedies included castor oil, animal bile and fats taken from many different kinds of animal. There is little on diagnosis, but the heart and pulse and arteries are described though in vague form by present-day standards. Diseases that are mentioned are those of fevers and infections and eye diseases. There would seem to be little advance on what was suspected to be the medical state of primitive Man. In some ways this is curious since there was the widespread practice of embalming, yet this inspired no great interest in anatomy or organ function.

The Old Testament mentions boils and plagues, largely as afflictions sent from God. Leviticus is full of rules of hygiene, some of which are sensible by present scientific standards and some of which seem simply to be superstitious and hallowed by tradition.

Despite the intrinsic interest of this ancient and primitive medicine, there does not seem to have been much progress in our terms. There were probably flashes of insight, but they were unrelated to any systematic body of knowledge and so did not attain significance. There must also have been some efficacious remedies, not excluding the supernatural invocations. The power of the mind and sincere belief in disease control and cure need no emphasis to any experienced practitioner of medicine. In older times there was probably much more susceptibility to suggestion than nowadays, and very much less scepticism about everything, perhaps therefore helping both patients and doctors, when definitely efficacious remedies were not available. Moreover, life expectancy was short—an index probably of the prevalence of disease—so that the inevitability of disease and death was apparent to all. This might very well have bred a certain stoicism and a hope for an after-life. The burial patterns of primitive Man and the embalming of bodies and massive monuments to the dead with all the appurtenances of travel beyond death suggest that this is so. This long-standing belief has many implications for medicine and how it is practised, especially near the point of death. If the belief should be culturally discarded, and there are some suggestive signs of this, the effect on medicine could be profound.

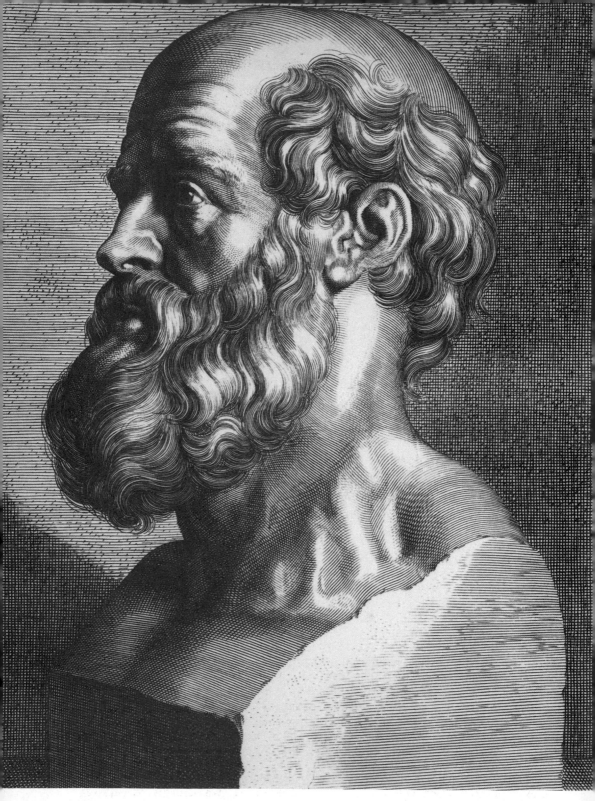

Hippocrates [460?–377?BC] (Reproduced by courtesy of the Wellcome Institute Library, London)

Chapter 2

The Greek tradition

The roots of western civilization and culture lie in the thoughts, philosophies and ideas of classical Greece. We still draw on them in general, even though the special and specific examples have greatly changed in the past 2500 years or so. Whitehead indeed has said that 'the European philosophical tradition is . . . a series of footnotes to Plato'. The major Greek philosophers raised all the great issues of life, living and death, most of which remain unanswered, yet they are still of relevance, not least in the practice of medicine. What the philosophers did establish, however, was a method of rational enquiry, which is the basis of science. In Greek times it was applied to morals, ethics, right action, and in seeking the meaning of virtue and justice and many other imponderable values for individuals and society. Yet the method showed that superficial appearance was not to be trusted, and that language had many ambiguities, and that even if a statement seemed to have clear meaning, close enquiry demonstrated that it had implications far beyond what had been first thought. The philosophers did not much check their speculations against verified and verifiable facts from nature. They looked inwards into their own natures and thoughts, rather than outwards to the world of nature. Yet they sensed a relationship with the universe and so with God, the gods, and the heavens, about all of which they speculated freely. There is a tendency nowadays, in science and medicine, to deplore and denigrate speculation, but there are times in history when there can be nothing else, since no other tools are available. And speculation is still an important feature of the higher reaches of scientific enquiry. Those who think otherwise delude themselves.

The Greek philosophical tradition began in Ionia, which is now the west-coast region in Turkey around Smyrna and including several of the islands close by. The mainland settlement was round three rivers, including the Maeander. What the intellectual conditions were for the beginnings of philosophy there is an intriguing question, but without a definite answer. What determines the rise of a centre of excellence, what maintains it over a period and why does its primacy fade? The answer lies somewhere in the hearts of men and the interplay of their minds and ideas, rather than in physical resources. Some groups sparkle and inspire their pupils to carry on their traditions; others remain humdrum and repetitive. This remains true for many institutions, not only medical.

Geographically Ionia was probably the recipient of two streams of cultural diffusion; one coming north along the Euphrates, and the other via Egypt and

Crete to the Greek mainland. The wars there drove some migrants eastwards across the sea to Ionia. Toynbee has suggested that some communities under stress from any source may be more likely to produce innovations. There needs, however, to be a fine balance between stress and leisure before intellectual advance can occur. The special interest of Ionia for medicine is that the island of Cos lies just to the south of it. It was there that Hippocrates, the Father of Medicine, was born in 460 BC and there that he practised. He must have been influenced by the thinking of Ionia and mainland Greece, for it is known that he travelled widely in both regions. He is, in fact, twice mentioned by Plato, so must have been well known to philosophers.

Socrates (c.470–399 BC) was particularly the one to introduce critical enquiry by dialogue, searching for meaning, for presuppositions behind any statement and for drawing out logical sequels from premisses. The analogies for science and medicine are obvious enough. Hippocrates (c.460 BC to c.377 BC) was contemporary with Socrates. Hippocrates has to be distinguished from the many who followed after him and probably made most of the contributions to the Hippocratic writings. These are probably the compilation of centuries, representing a tradition rather than just the work of one man. Yet Hippocrates was probably their inspiration and his personality, as that of any great teacher, pervades the written corpus. Socrates was often concerned with morality, ethics, the immortality of the soul and knowledge of the good. These were no doubt important for Hippocrates, and they remain so for medicine today. They determine how it shall be practised and with what aims and objectives.

The sciences of Hippocrates' time were astronomy, geometry and arithmetic, the last two owing advances to Pythagoras (580–498 BC). Plato (c.428–348 BC) followed Socrates in Athens, though he travelled to Egypt, Sicily and Italy. He recognized the sciences as arithmetic, plane and solid geometry, astronomy and harmonics.

Aristotle (384–324 BC) was a physician and a physician's son. He inherited the Socratic, Platonic and Hippocratic traditions, and was both physician and scientist as well as philosopher. He made direct observations on marine fauna, and in contemplating nature classified and dissected many animals and constructed a Scale of Being (*Scala Naturae*), though he did not visualize an evolutionary progression, a concept that had to wait for Darwin for fuller expression. Strangely he maintained that gentlemen should know the theory but not the practice of medicine. Perhaps it was he who introduced the class distinction between physicians and surgeons which lasted so long!

Because of his great influence he helped perpetuate the theory of disease in which there are four humours and four qualities (*Figure 2.1*). The humours were designated blood, phlegm, white bile and black bile, and people might therefore have sanguine, phlegmatic, choleric and melancholic temperaments. The four qualities were cold and hot, moist and dry. All matter was thought to consist of earth, air, fire and water. This triple bank of fours could be manipulated this way and that and has no significance now. But the salutary lesson to be learned is that it was believed and acted upon by the medical profession and others for nearly 2000 years, without being recognized as mumbo-jumbo and arrant nonsense. Yet the facts with which to destroy this theory were at hand for many centuries. It shows that no amount of appeal and exposure to fact will drive out error. Beliefs remain more powerful than fact, and scientists and doctors are as prey to unsound belief as any. Aristotle, the first real theoretical and practical scientist and a great and influential man, demonstrates this well. No one, not even a seminal genius, can

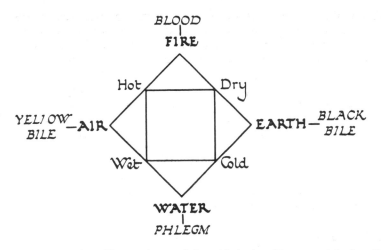

Figure 2.1 The four *Elements* in association with the four *Humors* and the four *Qualities*. (From *A Short History of Medicine*, 1928, reproduced by courtesy of Oxford University Press)

fully shake off all the intellectual accretions of his time. He recognized theoretical, practical and productive sciences. Mathematics and physics (natural science) were theoretical, ethics and politics were practical, and art and rhetoric (persuasion) were productive! At least this shows a very different outlook on life from the present day.

Little is known of the historical Hippocrates (460–377 BC) except that he was born and practised medicine on Cos, though he travelled to the neighbouring Greek mainland and to Asia Minor—the old Ionia. He and his followers are known more from the Hippocratic writings. On the island of Cos was a temple to Aesculapius (Asklepios), the god of healing. The sick, suffering and dying who repaired to the temple (Asklepieion) (*Figure 2.2*) were helped to sleep in the hope

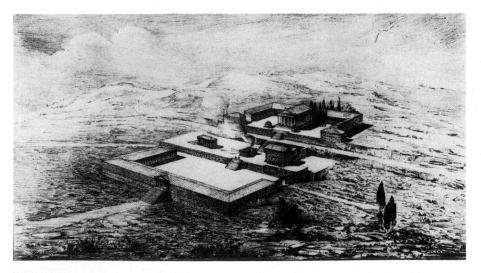

Figure 2.2 A reconstruction of the Asklepieion at Epidaurus in hellenistic times. (Reproduced by courtesy of the Wellcome Institute Library, London)

that in their dreams they would be visited by the god or gods and be shown how to get well. No doubt they were also physically cared for in pleasant surroundings with gardens, fountains and cool places, attended by what would now be seen to be nurses and doctors (Asclepiads). It was probably here that Hippocrates gained practical knowledge of medicine, for this he undoubtedly did have. Greece was also the home of education. Plato founded his Academy, Aristotle his Lyceum, and Hippocrates a school of medicine, for he was known to have a real concern for teaching. This may not have been bedside teaching but rather, in the way of the times, by discussion, disputation and dialogue. But it gave posterity the Hippocratic Writings.

It is not possible to do justice to the works of Hippocrates in a short book. He is especially famous for his Oath. There are several versions of this, but a representative one by a modern translator reads:

'I swear by Apollo the healer, by Aesculapius, by Health and all the powers of healing, and call to witness all the gods and goddesses that I may keep this Oath and Promise to the best of my ability and judgement.

'I will pay the same respect to my master in the Science as to my parents and share my life with him and pay all my debts to him. I will regard his sons as my brothers and teach them the Science, if they desire to learn it, without fee or contract.

'I will hand on precepts, lectures and all other learning to my sons, to those of my master and to those pupils duly apprenticed and sworn, and to none other.

'I will use my power to help the sick to the best of my ability and judgement; I will abstain from harming or wronging any man by it.

'I will not give a fatal draught to anyone if I am asked, nor will I suggest any such thing. Neither will I give a woman means to procure an abortion.

'I will be chaste and religious in my life and in my practice.

'I will not cut, even for the stone, but I will leave such procedures to the practitioners of that craft.

'Whenever I go into a house, I will go to help the sick and never with the intention of doing harm or injury. I will not abuse my position to indulge in sexual contacts with the bodies of women or of men, whether they be freemen or slaves.

'Whatever I see or hear, professionally or privately, which ought not to be divulged, I will keep secret and tell no one.

'If, therefore, I observe this Oath and do not violate it, may I prosper both in my life and in my profession, earning good repute among all men for all time. If I transgress and forswear this Oath, may my lot be otherwise.'

This is worth a little consideration. It is of interest in its appeal to deities, particularly those concerned with healing. Apollo was the first of these and others, including Aesculapius, came later, and the goddess of Health was Hygiea. There is a religious background to Hippocratic medicine.

There is reverence for teachers and something of a closed shop for medicine with preferential treatment for sons of doctors. This is not surprising. There were many quacks and charlatans in those days, and craft guilds have always been careful about those whom they are willing to admit to their mysteries. Medical students now have to be 'bona fide' and properly signed on by their medical schools.

The plain duty of the doctor not to harm or have the intention of doing so is very firmly stated. So the Oath is equally firm on euthanasia and procuring abortion. For over 2000 years this has been the guide, though in the 1980s the rightness of these attitudes is being called into question.

The decision not to perform surgery—cutting for bladder stone was one of the commonest operations of antiquity—is interesting because craft and handwork were not considered occupations fit for gentlemen. This attitude has persisted until well into the twentieth century and has still not entirely disappeared. This seeming divorce of hand from brain has probably been of detriment to the progress of medicine, though surgeons could easily agree that their craft should not be practised by physicians!

The matters of confidentiality and sexual abuse are still very much with us; in the first because of the immense modern complexity of storing information. In sexual abuse it is pertinent to note the reference both to slaves and to freemen. The real problem is that the doctor is often in a position of moral authority and can exert undue influence on the behaviour of patients. In modern form this highlights the dilemma of doctors caring for prisoners, not in any matter of sexual abuse, but in possibly condoning, aiding and abetting in punishment. Moreover, in occupational medicine both doctor and patient have allegiances to the company for which they each work, which may conflict with the simple one-to-one relationship, which is the paradigm for most of clinical medicine.

There need perhaps be little wonder that the Oath has persisted for so long. It embodies much of the best traditions of medicine and how doctors should behave towards their patients. It is no longer formally administered to new medical graduates as it used to be. Yet its traditions pervade the whole of medical practice and these rub off on to students, so that they conform with the spirit of the Oath, even when they do not know nor swear to its exact content. Because there is much anxiety about the conduct of some doctors, especially in using psychiatric techniques on those imprisoned by the State, often for political reasons, the World Medical Association has produced a modern version of the Hippocratic Oath to meet present conditions. It was done in a Declaration of Geneva in 1948, which was brought up to date at Sydney in 1968. This shows that the principles enunciated by Hippocrates are still of importance.

Further writings are on good behaviour and right actions and characteristics of students and doctors, but what catches the clinical eye is the series of careful case notes of patients. This is the first instance of acute observation with careful recording. Many of the cases appear in *Epidemics*, which describes fevers and their outcome, which was often death. The characteristics of the fevers, the nature of the stool and urine, the appearance of the face, twitchings, convulsions and coma are all described day by day. And often some background is given as to where the patient normally lived and what he did.

Another remarkable work is that of *Airs, Waters, Places*. This is an effort to relate the environment and climate to the health, disease, cure or worsening of a patient. Also considered is the constitution of the patient, a somewhat nebulous concept, yet denoting in some individuals a certain proneness to certain sorts of disease. This seems a real enough problem which advances in science might ultimately be able to answer in genetic and biochemical terms.

Prognosis is fascinating for its emphasis on the art of prediction. It is in fact a most valuable asset for the practitioner, especially when, as in those days, there were no specific remedies. The doctor himself, the relatives and friends, and perhaps even the patient himself wish to know the likely outcome, and especially whether that will be life or death.

In various *Regimens* treatment is described. They consisted mainly of some doubtfully efficacious drugs and herbal remedies and of what can only be described as hopeful manipulations of the diet. It is interesting to note how perennial this is. There is much crankiness about diet in medicine. It stems from a vague belief that what you eat is what you are. It is interesting to see how old that belief is and that it is still active.

Aphorisms is famous. It starts, 'Life is short, science is long; opportunity is elusive, experiment dangerous, judgement is difficult.' A slightly less prosaic version is, 'Life is short, the Art long, opportunity fleeting, experience fallacious, judgement difficult.' Science is often translated as art. There was in fact no real difference between them in those early times. The advice in the *Aphorisms* is clinical and homiletic. For instance there is the one, 'Desperate cases need the most desperate remedies.' And also such as, 'Starchy food is most difficult to digest in summer and autumn, easiest in winter and next easiest in spring.' There are magnificent insights alongside extreme banalities and useless advice. It is like this throughout medical history.

Fractures is excellent for its time, showing, as might be expected from such a source, sound common sense. It recognizes simple and compound fractures, and dislocations. There are descriptions of how to reduce them, and on the use of slings, splints and bandages. The poor prognosis of compound fractures is known.

The Seed and the Nature of the Child discusses conception and the growth of the fetus. The view was that male seed and female seed are mixed together in the womb. The author describes what he saw in an early abortion, and although no part is named it is fairly obvious that the specimen consisted of amnion, chorion, blood and embryo, as they came to be called later.

The Heart is a sort of anatomical treatise. Auricles, ventricles, valves, vessels and the pericardium are seen, though not named and much of the observation is inaccurate. This is because the underlying ideas of the function and nutrition of the heart carried the observer away from simple observation into the realms of interpretation in terms of what he believed. The error persists in us all, and has not been cast out with the passage of time.

There are many other books within the Hippocratic canon, and each has its own fascination, in giving insight into the medical mind and its methods of more than 2000 years ago. In some ways we are now in a very different world, light years away from classical Greece, and in other ways we have scarcely moved. Looked at critically, Grecian medicine was very little advanced on primitive medicine in practice. Some surgery of trauma was probably efficacious, but practical medicine was still essentially nursing care with some change in diet, and perhaps a few drugs which might or might not have been of value. Yet the theoretical base, ultimately to prove so fruitful, had changed from the primitive beyond all recognition. Science had started. There was a rational method of enquiry. Discussion was free and encouraged. Classification of phenomena had begun—an essential part of science, at least until it can become more completely mathematical. There was observation and careful recording of data, and in the hands of Aristotle even some beginnings of experiment in dissection. The seeds of progress were sown, even though the significance of the sowing would not have been comprehended at the time.

The medical profession, as specialists, was established too. It had a corpus of knowledge exemplified by Hippocrates. It had to have appeals to the supernatural, but the natural, in terms of observation, recording and rational further enquiry, was now part of medicine and of science.

The campaigns of Alexander the Great carried the Greek empire far and wide, eastwards to Afghanistan and southwards through Syria to Egypt, where Alexandria was founded in 322 BC. His tutor as a boy in Macedonia was Aristotle. Perhaps as a result of this Alexander always carried with his armies and colonizers, scientists and philosophers, among them what we would now call doctors. At Alexandria a flourishing medical school was founded, and ultimately the Hippocratic library of Cos was consigned to the renowned library of the city, whose burning by Christian zealots deprived the world of a priceless collection. For a very brief time the ban on dissection of the human body was lifted in Alexandria, which was unusual in the Hellenic world. Herophilus and Erasistratus, both born about 300 BC, took advantage of this; and the first of them described venous sinuses in the brain, especially the confluence of some of them in the torcula Herophili (the winepress of Herophilus). He also described the duodenum as being twelve finger-breadths in length, hence the present name. He counted the pulse rate by a clock. Erasistratus distinguished the cerebrum (upper part of the brain) from the cerebellum (lower part concerned with balance) and saw the difference between motor and sensory nerves, for the two varieties enter the spinal cord separately. Not surprisingly, these two physicians did not always distinguish between nerves, veins and arteries and tendons in the limbs.

In Alexandria there was some scepticism about the doctrine of the four humours, as accepted by Hippocrates and Aristotle. Erasistratus attributed disease to an excessive amount of blood in the parts, or plethora. A major theory was that air entered the lungs and then went to the heart, where it was changed into a Vital Spirit which was carried to all the body through the arteries. It is sad that so little remains of the work of these Alexandrians because of the incendiarists. The Greek tradition which they picked up, and then sustained and increased, passed almost imperceptibly towards Rome. The power of Rome rose and that of Greece declined, and as we have seen medicine tends to follow in the wake of progress in other fields, particularly those of conquest and flourishing economics and safe, sound politics. It seems to be an art of civilization, flourishing best when that is well founded.

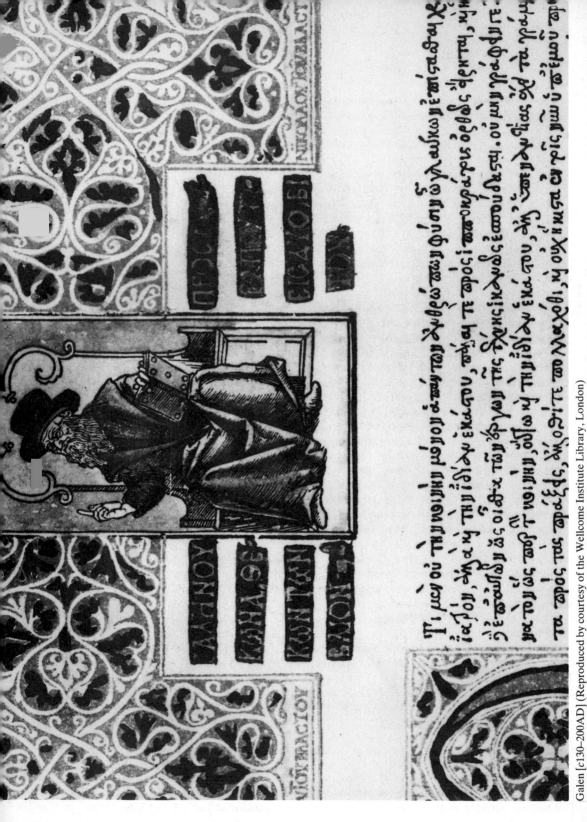

Galen [c130–200AD] (Reproduced by courtesy of the Wellcome Institute Library, London)

18

Chapter 3

Roman times

The dominance of Rome extends from about the first century BC until about AD 500. Along with much of the western world, Egypt was taken into the Roman Empire. By then the medical school of Alexandria had greatly faded; or at least there is nothing surviving to show otherwise, because of the destruction of the library of nearly three-quarters of a million volumes. The centre for medicine therefore shifted to the capital of Rome during the first century BC. At that time there were no doctors as such in Rome. Each householder was his own physician and cared for his family and slaves, appealing to the vast array of gods, of which there was one for almost every state of disease and for every house and social function. Greek doctors moved in, bringing their expertise with them and for sale. Sicily and Southern Italy were still much under Greek influence. The doctors received a mixed welcome, being approved by some and abhorred by others. In general, however, their status slowly improved.

The first of the Greek physicians in Rome was Asclepiades of Bithynia (124 BC). He was a worthy forerunner of a long tradition. He did not follow Hippocrates in the belief that disease was caused by imbalance of the four humours, but introduced his own notion that disease was caused by various combinations of contraction and relaxation of particles of the body. Similar theories keep cropping up throughout history. We are still told to tone ourselves up, or relax when we are tense. Asclepiades taught a small body of disciples.

In AD 30 Celsus (*Figure 3.1*) published his work *De Re Medicina*. He was not a doctor, so this is essentially a compilation based mainly on the Hippocratic Writings, and adopting their high moral tone with sensible recommendations. He adopts the disease theory of Asclepiades, but unlike him does not advocate an active attack on disease, but with Hippocrates is willing to wait a little for 'the healing force of nature' (*Vis Medicatrix Naturae*) to do its benign work. The two types of doctor have existed through time—activists and passivists. Sometimes one is needed and sometimes the other.

In medical treatment there were only changes of diet, some drugs and baths (both cold and hot) to be prescribed. Asclepiades may have been the originator of the Roman penchant for bathing. But in surgery Celsus writes of plastic operations for restoration of the nose, of cutting for stone, and removing goitres and the tonsils, as well as repairing hernias. Surgical instruments of the time included forceps, trocars and cannulae, and specula of various kinds. That the book

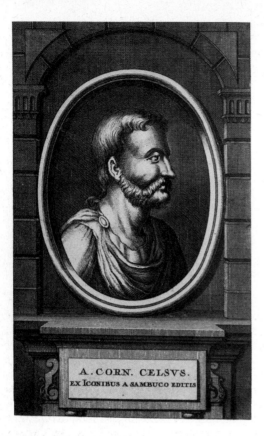

A . CORN. CELSVS.
EX ICONIBUS A SAMBUCO EDITIS

Figure 3.1 A. Cornelius Celsus [1st century AD]. (Reproduced by courtesy of the Wellcome Institute Library, London)

contained much contemporary wisdom is also attested by the fact that it was re-published in Florence in 1478, and went into many further editions. But this also shows how little medicine had advanced over 14 centuries.

There were other Greek surgeons about the time of Celsus, and a matter of some interest is that they applied ligatures to arterial aneurysms (swellings), an operation that engaged the attention of John Hunter in the eighteenth century.

Soranus of Ephesus flourished in the second century AD and his work was on pregnancy, childbirth, gynaecology (diseases peculiar to women) and children (*Figure 3.2*). His main claim to later fame is that he advocated turning the child round in the womb in certain cases of difficult labour. This was done by inserting the whole hand through the vagina and into the uterus, pushing up the baby's head and then pulling on a foot and leg. The operation is called internal version. It was revived by Paré in the sixteenth century. It has a long and honourable history of much value to childbearing women, though now it is very rarely used in advanced countries. Other, safer techniques have superseded it.

The towering figure of the Roman period was Galen (AD 131–201). He was a 'know-all', with an answer for everything. His writing output was prodigious; some attribute 500 books to him. With this cocksureness, overwhelming wordiness and few opponents his place in medical history would be secure. But more important for his legend was his belief that the body is simply a vehicle for the soul. Following

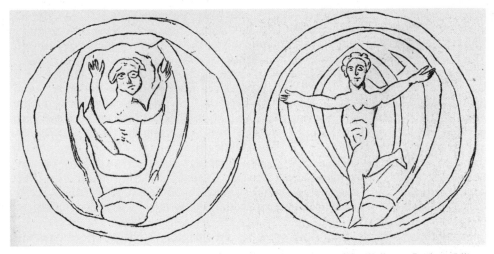

Figure 3.2 Fetus *in utero* from a Soranus MS. (Reproduced by courtesy of the Wellcome Institute Library, London)

Aristotle he believed that everything had its function determined by God, and he was therefore a teleologist, i.e. he believed that structures are designed for a specific end. With this sort of doctrine of the body exemplifying the Creator's purpose and design he had an obvious appeal for both Christian and Islamic faiths which dominated the centuries after the fall of Rome.

Galen was born in Pergamum, and he studied anatomy at Smyrna, and later in Alexandria where he saw and handled a human skeleton. It is interesting to observe the continuing importance for about 600 years of Ionia and Egypt in medicine. But during his lifetime dissection of the human was not permitted, so his knowledge of anatomy was derived mainly from the pig, dog and Barbary ape. This was obviously good work, but too vast an edifice of guesswork and speculation was built on these inadequate foundations. After Alexandria he was soon in Rome where he practised successfully, but he also travelled back to Pergamum and into Sicily and Greece. In practice he followed Hippocrates in deriving everything from the four humours, and it was Galen who drew these out into the temperaments of sanguine, phlegmatic, choleric and melancholic. His armamentarium was, as before his time, that of diet, a few drugs and bathing. Possibly he excelled in diagnosis and prognosis, and many reputations have been built on these alone. However, Galen does not record case histories in the Hippocratic way.

In anatomy Galen was quite good on bones and joints, though he did not name them well. And he knew about muscles from his dissections of the Barbary ape. His knowledge of the brain was good too. He recognized seven cranial nerves (there are 12), the meninges surrounding the brain, and many structures in the brain, such as the hemispheres, cerebellum, ventricles and corpus callosum. Experimentally on pigs he knew that cutting the spinal cord resulted in paralysis below the lesion, and he also knew that injury to the right side of the cerebrum caused disorder on the opposite side of the body. This is all remarkable, but then he misled subsequent centuries with his physiological theories.

The theories held sway for many centuries, so are worth a word. A spirit (*pneuma*) is taken in with each breath. It comes from the general world-spirit.

From the lungs it passes to the heart through the pulmonary vein(s). In the left ventricle the *pneuma* meets the blood, which is made in the liver from chyle, made from the digestion of food in the gut and transported to the liver by the portal vein. The liver imbues the chyle with *Natural Spirit*. This passes to the right ventricle and on to the lungs where it is exhaled. But a little of this mixture from the liver seeps through the ventricular wall into the left ventricle, where mixing with the *pneuma* it forms *Vital Spirit*. The action of the heart causes ebb and flow in both veins and arteries, there being then no notion of circulation. That blood reaching the brain has added to it the *Animal Spirit* or soul. This is carried by the supposedly hollow nerves to all parts of the body, imbuing them with movement and sensation. In some form or another these notions keep appearing. By present standards they are nonsense and simply show the results, usually of no value or even counterproductive, of raising too much theory and hypothesis on too little observed fact. In many fields the imagination should soar, but in the practical art of medicine it may be misleading.

From these various authors it can be seen that the Roman period showed a further working out of the Greek tradition in a different setting. Roman ideas *per se* added virtually nothing. Yet because of the orderly mind and military prowess Rome contributed much in general hygiene, in sanitation, in building sewers and in warming houses. There were the great aqueducts bringing clean water, and the Cloaca Maxima discharging sewage from Rome. Bathing, both public and private, was almost a religious ritual. Hypocausts were the first forms of central heating in houses and in military garrisons. Sanitary engineering has made enormous contributions to the public health, largely by empirical methods, not necessarily guided by sound science. Yet that is the way of many things found to be valuable. The practical men get on with the job. Good results accrue, and then scientiests later explain why this was so. There is a place for many varieties of enterprise. Superiority of one over another can rarely be properly claimed. The history of science and of medicine ought to breed much humility among their present practitioners, lest they might fall into ancient errors.

The Romans might also be thought to be the founders of the idea of hospitals, though their forerunners could very well be the Asklepieia of Greece. But on the Tiber near Rome there was a small island to which sick and dying slaves were sent. If they survived they were set free. Efforts were therefore made to help and cure them, probably by other slaves. It was this class that practised medicine before the coming of the Greek physicians, for no Roman citizen would demean himself by being active in medicine or surgery. The navy and the army, however, had to have their surgeons. They were trained in Rome and other centres, and in the early days of the empire they held a non-commissioned rank, and were definitely much subordinate to the combatant officers. Yet later their status rose, and it is of interest that they were exempt from taxes and from combatant duty, this last remaining until the present day. Physicians had a higher status than surgeons and often took part in government. Even more unusual is it to find that cities sometimes appointed physicians on a salary to care for the sick poor. A Government-provided service of some kind is an ancient idea, and has been sporadically implemented through the ages. And as the legions marched through Europe they established their forts and garrisons, in which there were often hospitals of a kind, mainly for dealing with injuries.

The decline and fall of the Roman Empire is a fascinating story, told in glorious style by one of the most famous historians. For this present more mundane purpose it needs only to be noted that the Emperor Constantine, the first Christian emperor, moved his capital in AD 330 from Rome to Byzantium, which then became Constantinople, and later Istanbul. One of the reasons for the move—subsidiary perhaps to political, military, economic and social factors—may have been the prevalence of disease causing death in large numbers. The influence of such diseases as malaria, plague and typhus, and of typhoid and dysentery in fighting troops is not as widely known as it should be. There is a role for medicine and sanitary engineering in shoring up civilizations and in winning wars, by preventing widespread disease, and nowadays curing it rapidly when epidemic infections occur. With the move to Byzantium the centre of influence, including that of medicine, also changed. Orthodox Christianity and Islam added powerfully to that influence, as will be seen.

A glance back through this period of about 600 years shows a mass of useless theory, built on humours, vitalism or tone, and yet some pragmatic practical approaches in surgery, obstetrics and sanitary engineering, and possibly even personal hygiene. Military surgery was well advanced, and alcohol and mandragora were used as primitive anaesthetics. But physicians still had to be content with diagnosis and prognosis with pontifications about diet, useless drugs with few exceptions, warmth, cold, bathing, rest and sleep. The *vis medicatrix naturae*, with a fortunate reluctance to interfere actively, kept them in their estate as gentlemen, whose interests were scholarly and patrician.

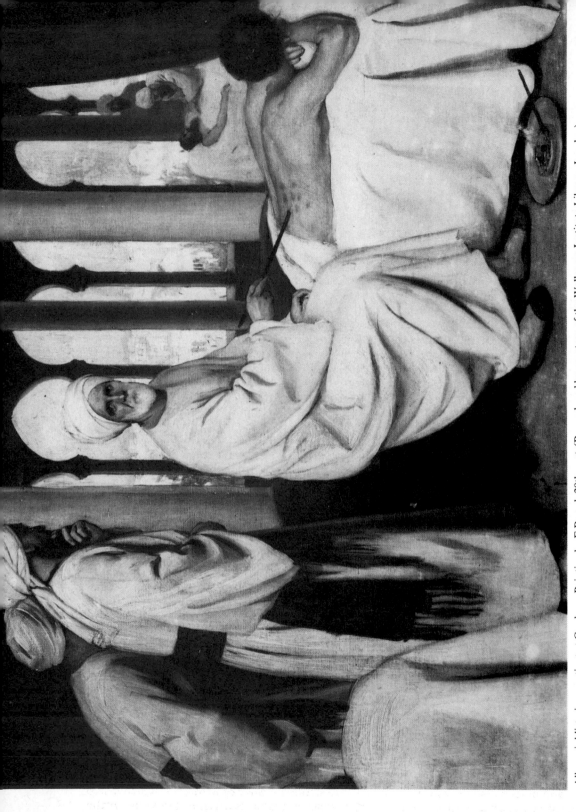

Albucasis blistering a patient at Cordova. Painting by E Board, 20th cent (Reproduced by courtesy of the Wellcome Institute Library, London)

Chapter 4

The Arabian contribution

The Greek and Roman traditions in medicine were obviously not limited to natives of those two countries. Ideas are not confined within geographical boundaries. They diffuse in many directions. The same is true of the Arabian contribution. It was inherited, used and added to by all the nationalities and sects who came under the influence of the Byzantine Empire and the teachings of Islam. This influence, like that of Greece and Rome, spread far along the shores of the Mediterranean, along both northern and southern littorals. Geographically therefore, all the cultures are to be thought of as including Asia Minor, Greece, Italy, Sicily and the Iberian Peninsula, as well as Egypt and the north coast of Africa to Tunis and Morocco. The special feature of this period is the use of the Arabic language as the cultural vehicle, though a variety of peoples took part in the ideas and practices of the time, and among them were Jews, Arabs, Christians and Muslims. In the history of ideas there are no monopolies by creed, nationality or any other of the usually artificial divisions of mankind.

In contrast with a common concept of the Byzantines, many of the emperors and caliphs were patrons, supporters and promoters of the arts and intellectual activities. They gathered around them scholars and books. It was the translation of these from Greek especially, but also Latin that kept medicine alive at this period.

In AD 431 the patriarch of Jerusalem, Nestorius, was banished because of the heresy he propounded that Christ had relatively independent natures, human and divine. This made Mary the mother of Jesus and not the mother of God. The result was that Nestorius and his followers emigrated to Edessa in Asia Minor and there they set up a school of medicine, and later they moved south-west into Persia (Iran) and started other schools. These Christians translated the ancient Greek medical texts into Arabic.

Mohammed was born in AD 570 and the Islamic influence rose immensely in the seventh century and after. One of its great physicians was Rhazes (860–932), who worked in Persia and Baghdad. He wrote voluminously in Arabic and was the first to distinguish between smallpox and measles. In his books he cites the older authors and then gives his own views. In the Hippocratic tradition he gives case records.

Avicenna (980–1037) was the most famous of Arab physicians. He was Persian and practised mainly in that country. He wrote a *Canon of Medicine*, which lasted for centuries as a medical text, albeit translated later into Latin. He knew of the works of Aristotle and Galen, and was an acute clinical observer who often put his thoughts into aphorisms.

In surgery the fame of this period belongs to the Moor, Albucasis (936–1013), who was born in Cordoba in Spain and practised there. The city was large and a centre of learning, with a large library and many hospitals. The surgery was still crude, concerned mainly with trauma and the opening of abscesses, with some eye surgery, and heavy-handed manipulation of spinal deformities, which must often have caused great damage. He advocated and used the actual red-hot cautery in stopping bleeding.

It remains only to mention the names of Avenzoar (1072–1162), Averroes (1126–1198) and the Jew Maimonides (1135–1204) (*Figure 4.1*), all of Spain, though Maimonides later moved to Cairo because he would not adopt the Muslim faith. These all upheld the tenets of the best medical practice and wrote, often wisely in our terms, so that a medical heritage from Greece, Rome and Arabia was maintained. But the Moslem Empire fell in the thirteenth century just as previous ones had. It had improved the study of mathematics with algebra and had helped with the development of chemistry through alchemy. This sought the philosopher's stone which would transmute base metals into gold, but in the search some valuable

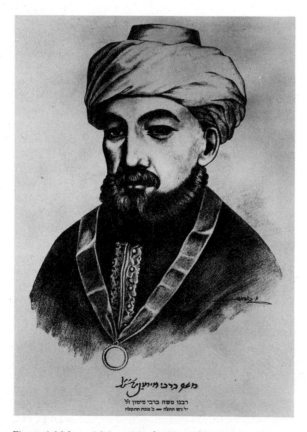

רבנו משה ברבי מימון זצ׳
יר נש תתלה — כ טבת תתקסה

Figure 4.1 Moses Maimonides [1135–1204]. (Reproduced by courtesy of the Wellcome Institute Library, London)

observations of nature were made. There are many wrong-headed pursuits that contain a germ of truth within them.

It is worth note that 16 or 17 centuries elapsed from the time of Hippocrates to the decline of Arabian medicine, yet it is difficult to discern much progress except in a very few isolated instances. There were ideas in plenty but no method by which to put them to the test rigorously and no valuable technology to be borrowed from other disciplines for use in medicine. It could not be otherwise at the time. Progress is seldom linearly upwards. There are plateaus and undulations upwards and downwards as well as definite regress. It is quite an achievement to hold to the plateau, and that is what Arabian medicine did.

Drawing by Leonardo da Vinci, at Windsor (Royal Library). (Reproduced by courtesy of the Wellcome Institute Library, London)

Chapter 5

The Middle Ages

The exact period to be called the Middle Ages is disputed but for the present will be taken to run from about AD 400 to 1500, that is from the decline of Rome to the stirrings of the Renaissance. However, ideas, their growth, waning or stagnation are not to be confined by dates, as already emphasized.

In medicine the Middle Ages are dull. A few bright lights dispel the darkness fitfully. And yet in general we have to be grateful that much was not entirely lost. It was a time for holding the line rather than advancing or retreating. There was little innovation as scholars of the church picked over the bones of the works of classical antiquity, and those of Galen, commenting on them and amending them in translation without any notion of testing them for their truth or otherwise. Indeed it was the curse of the time to accept that they were true. This was an age of scholasticism with a general presupposition that everything worth while had been discovered and committed to posterity in books. The duty of the scholars was therefore to read, mark, learn and inwardly digest these old works and preserve them more or less intact. This partly explains the long and continuing influence of Galen. His opinions were firmly stated, even when they were wrong, and so he was an authority for clergy of the scholastic kind. He had a philosophy of body, mind and soul, which was highly acceptable to the religion of the developing church.

It was an Age of Faith, from which the scholasticism sprang. The church held great sway during all these years. In Europe the elements forming society were those of classical antiquity, the Roman inheritance, the social forms of the largely Vandal invaders from the north and above all the church. It was the clergy who had the monopoly of knowledge and education. It was they who had access to libraries and they could read and write. Moreover, they were able to do this in the common language of Latin. Everywhere they could communicate with one another. Because of these educational attributes they were in demand everywhere, for they were needed as civil servants for the myriad governments of the day, in the drafting of policies, treaties and agreements, in handling financial affairs, in negotiations as well as in interpreting the law. The clergy stepped into all these breaches in the social structure, since there was no one else capable of doing so. It was a vast achievement bringing a sort of unity throughout Europe which perhaps has never been seen since. Not only were they in large measure controllers and advisers on secular affairs, they claimed and were accorded almost total spiritual power. The

Pope and the church he led and commanded were indeed a force to be reckoned with in human affairs in the West.

Revelation, pure reason, dogma, theological dispute and arid commentaries on ancient texts are not a suitable environment for the flourishing of science and practical medicine. Moreover, the religious beliefs of the time tended to be that disease was a punishment for sin, and that life was a fraught journey to be endured until death should lead to the bliss of an after-life. It can be seen that this is no philosophy on which to build a system of medical practice designed to prevent disease and death in individuals, and interfering with God's purposes. This shows what is often forgotten in present-day practice, that perceptions of what medicine is, what it should do and how it does it are totally dependent on the general climate of opinion of the times. It has no totally independent autonomy from the general ideas of its period. A presently obvious phenomenon, occasioned by medical mobility, is that the practice of medicine varies much to accord with its surrounding culture. The aims and objectives for medicine vary in time and place and there is still not sufficient careful analysis of the cultural factors in the western world that affect the practice of medicine and what its aims should be.

Despite the church's philosophy being a cause of nihilism in medicine, it did reinforce one of the pillars of both Christianity and medicine—the belief in the importance of each individual in the sight of God. From the earliest times the doctors had cared for patients without concern for colour, class or creed. In the Middle Ages, however, there was religious backing for this previously humanistic belief. It is one of the great ideas of history, with value not only in medicine, but in the shaping of societies and their politics and so in the destruction of dictatorships and monopolies and corporate oppressive movements of all kinds.

Not only in this idea was the church helpful to medicine, it was also practical in caring for the sick in infirmaries attached to abbeys, convents, priories and cathedrals. Here there was nursing care with warmth, food, shelter and prayer supplemented by herbs, and concoctions made from them, from the monastery garden. In the present-day rush to find specific remedies for every ill these non-specific backgrounds of care of the sick are not to be demeaned. They are desired by the ailing person who needs to feel important and loved, and to be tended with compassion. And the effect of such caring on those who give it is not to be forgotten, for it may frequently be elevating emotionally and spiritually. In London the religious foundations of St. Bartholomew's Hospital (1123) and St. Thomas's Hospital (1215) began in this period.

This mediaeval time has some strange admixtures. Naturally there were many saints associated with healing, but the most famous were the Arab Christians, Saints Cosmas and Damian (*Figure 5.1*). They were credited with miraculous cures, especially in surgery. There is a famous picture of them in which the leg of a white man has been amputated and then replaced with one from a black man—perhaps one of the earliest depictions of transplantation. It is interesting to recall the outcry among some sections when in the mid-twentieth century a black man's heart was transplanted into a white man in South Africa!

Dating from this time were St. Vitus, whose name is associated with the uncontrollable movements of chorea, a form of rheumatism, as in a continued dance, and St. Anthony, whose Fire is variously thought to be erysipelas, which is a very red skin rash, or ergotism. The latter is most likely. Ergot is a fungus that grows on rye which was much used in making bread. Active principles in ergot cause contraction of blood vessels in the limbs with agonizing pain and later

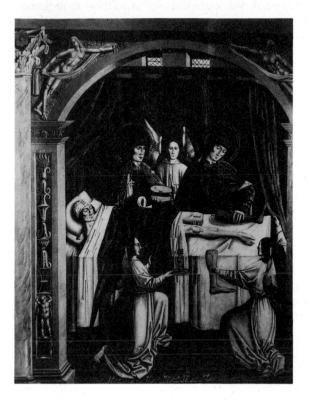

Figure 5.1 Saints Cosmas and Damian performing the miracle of the transplanted leg. Oil painting by Alonso de Sedano, Biergos, *c.* 1500. (Reproduced by courtesy of the Wellcome Institute Library, London)

gangrene. In women it causes contractions of the womb, which if pregnant may abort. In later centuries this observation was used to help women in labour by making the uterus contract after the birth of the baby to prevent haemorrhage.

The several other saints canonized for their healing powers are of little interest now. The real academic contribution of the church was in the keeping and translation of the older works, written in Greek, Syriac, and Arabic. The rendering of these in the *lingua franca* of Latin so that they became available to the intellectual world of the time and for many centuries later was a singular service which should not be underestimated. The scholar clerics maintained the life of the Greek, Roman and Arabian traditions in medicine, even if they added little to practice and nothing to the science. With the preoccupations of that thousand years and more—inimical as they were to the advance of medicine and science, because of the more major pursuits of scholasticism, theology, religion and faith—it is a matter for thankfulness that much more was not lost.

Every civilization carries within it the seeds of its own destruction. Those seeds are ideas which slowly grow in opposition to the prevailing ones, which are often simply accepted presuppositions and are unquestioned. The ideas generate actions, whose significance at first is not recognized, but ultimately the nature of society is transformed. The Middle Ages gradually gave way to the Renaissance partly because of undiscerned opposition to the church, its teaching and virtual monopoly of education.

The first universities were in fact founded to further the education of monks and priests beyond that of the monastic and other church schools. But in addition there came wandering lay scholars from all over Europe, who gathered together in their national sects at first, and somewhat informally latched on to the teachings of the university. The first universities were those of Paris (1110), Bologna (1158), Oxford (1167), Montpellier (1181), Cambridge (1209), Padua (1222), Naples (1224), and there were many others mainly in the southern half of Europe in Italy, Switzerland, France and Spain. Many of them took to teaching medicine though often of a very theoretical kind; and as always, based on the work of the old masters.

Most of the mediaeval universities started with faculties of theology and law, as might be expected. With medicine these three remained the major faculties for many centuries (*Figure 5.2*). And medicine is not to be thought of only as the sort of study we know now. It embraced much of what was science, so that doctors of those times were definitely polymaths. But one of the remarkable phenomena of the age was the medical school of Salerno on Italy's west coast, just south of Naples. In some aspects it was centuries ahead of its time, and yet it has disappeared without trace. Although it was close to the Benedictine monastery of Monte

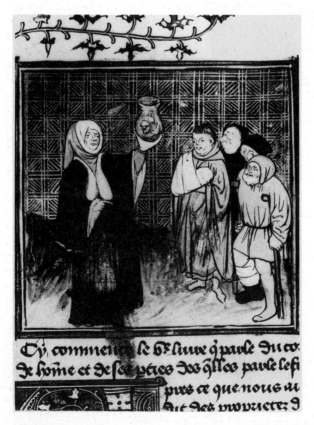

Figure 5.2 Physician examining urine flask. From a MS in the Bibliothèque Nationale, Paris. (Reproduced by courtesy of the Wellcome Institute Library, London)

Cassino, it seems to have owed nothing to the church at all, but was a lay foundation. This is some evidence of the quiet forces growing in opposition to the relative monopoly of the church. However, it is recorded that relations between the doctors of Salerno and the monks were cordial. The school flourished from about 1100 to 1300. Its founding is somewhat in dispute and lost in the charming legend that it started as the result of the coming together of a Jew, an Arab, a Greek and a Latin. Whether or not this is fact, there can be no doubt that the place was in a strategic position to pick up Greek, Arabic, Roman and Jewish cultural and medical influences. It has earlier been stressed that each culture spread along the Mediterranean littoral and one of the pivotal areas of each was in Sicily and southern Italy.

Astonishing is the fact that women were taught medicine at Salerno and were also on the staff. Obstetrics was certainly practised there by Trotula, and she wrote a book on the subject about AD 1050. Human dissection was not allowed, but anatomy was studied from the pig, and the *Anatomia Porci* by Kopho of the school was the first textbook of anatomy. The school was first under the aegis of King Roger II of Sicily and later of Emperor Frederick II. In 1221 the emperor decreed that no one should practise medicine unless he had been duly examined by the masters of Salerno. Moreover, entrants to the school were required to have spent time in the study of logic and be not less than 21 years of age. The medical course lasted 5 years and was completed by an examination and the swearing of an oath. All this has a strangely modern ring, for the medical undergraduate course still lasts for 5 years, and there is a minimum age of entry, which is now usually 18, but there are still those who call for a more general education prior to beginning the study of medicine. And there seem to have been no restrictions on entry to Salerno based on sex, colour, class or creed. Why the school should have gone into decline is baffling, when it was so enlightened and progressive.

The famous publication of the school was the *Regimen Sanitatis Salernitanum* which ran to about 300 editions up to the mid-nineteenth century. It consists of several hundred verses with advice on the maintenance of health by diet, rest, sleep, exercise, the use of herbal remedies and moderation in all things. It reads like a *Complete Home Doctor*, and perhaps that is just how it was used.

As the light of Salerno dimmed, that of Montpellier in medical education glowed more brightly. There is no certainty as to why, but situated on the coast in southern France, almost midway between Sicily and Spain, it presumably came under the old Greek, Roman and Arabian influences. The medical school flourished particularly in the thirteenth and fourteenth centuries in the Middle Ages. It was visited by many renowned doctors from all over Europe, and some were students there. John of Gaddesden (1280–1361) was an English student who became professor of medicine at Oxford. A Portuguese native, Petrus Hispanus, who studied at Montpellier and became a physician, was elected Pope John XXI. Guy de Chauliac (1300–1367), a Frenchman, was also a student, and ultimately a remarkable surgeon, who published *Chirurgia Magna*. This was clear and concise and, although recounting some history, included original observations. He operated on hernias and deplored the sacrifice of the testis at operation, and he also advocated trusses. He 'cut for stone' in the bladder using the the usual route through the perineum. He used weights over pulleys to maintain traction on fractured bones of the leg, a method still used today. And he introduced the rope attached to a beam over the bed of a patient by which he could heave himself up the bed, and this simple device must by now have been a boon to millions.

Another mediaeval medical school was that of Bologna (1158) in Northern Italy. It is not far from Padua which followed it 64 years later in founding a university in 1222. This is one of the early hints of the migration northwards of intellectual activity in medicine. It had ebbed and flowed essentially round the Mediterranean basin, but after the Renaissance it moved steadily northwards, though this generalization overlooks the importance of Paris, Amsterdam, Oxford and other centres. Yet the generalization is essentially correct.

At Bologna, Thaddeus the Florentine (1223–1303), also known as Taddeo Alderotti, introduced clinical teaching and discussions of clinical cases. Still, however, the teaching apparently considered symptoms, prognosis and treatment; and the only physical signs of disease came from inspection of the patient and his effluxions of faeces, urine, vomit and sputum and other discharges.

Theodoric of Lucca (1205–1298) introduced a sponge in which were mandragora and opium. When soaked in hot water this was inhaled or swallowed by the patient. Undoubtedly, it could have had a powerful effect in deadening pain and indeed in inducing anaesthesia. Both mandrake and opium had been known since early times, and opium had been advocated for pain-killing in the heyday of Alexandria, by Heraclides of Tarentum (*fl.* second century AD).

It was at Bologna that the study of anatomy seriously began. Mundinus (*c.*1275–1326) wrote a textbook on the subject in 1316, and much of it was based on human dissection which was now increasingly allowed. The book still perpetuated much of Galen's teaching derived from animals, demonstrating how difficult it can be to shake off ideas and observations from the past. Slowly, it seems, the dead human body had become less sacrosanct in the eyes of the church and the public. For some time during the Middle Ages occasional post-mortem examinations had been held in public as a means of trying to establish the cause of death. But such autopsies were very perfunctory and did not include the limbs. There had also been the practice of occasional public dissection of executed criminals. This was carried out by a servant under the direction of a master who did not soil his hands, but read from a book as he sat raised on a dais above the proceedings. The demonstration therefore was mainly to confirm what was in the book, and was not used as a vehicle for novel observation. The birth of science in medicine was based on anatomical studies, and these began in earnest at Padua—as it were just up the road from Bologna—but almost 250 years later. Mundinus, however, may be credited with the fact that he undertook some of the dissections himself, so at least gaining some first-hand experience which readers from the book did not.

Other contributors to knowledge of anatomy, the artists, were often much more advanced than the doctors. The anatomical drawings of Leonardo da Vinci (1452–1519) are well known and are remarkably accurate in the depiction of muscles and bones and some of the vasculature and nerves.

There is that superb picture of the fetus in the womb also, and all of the drawings seem to show an intimate acquaintance with the subject which could probably only have come from careful and personal dissection. Yet these contributions made little effect on the medical fraternity. No doubt this was partly because there is usually poor communication across disciplines, a matter of serious significance down the centuries and persisting still, so that the doctors would not see the relevance of the artist's interest to their own work. Moreover, even if the doctors did know of this detailed anatomy, it was of little practical use to them. The value of basic sciences to medicine lies in having technology that can use them. Pure science gives an understanding of the world. Applied science uses that understanding. About the turn of the fourteenth century anatomy was pure science, and it had to wait for many decades before it became applied.

The power of medicine was negligible to cope with the ravages of epidemic infections in the Middle Ages. The worst of these was the Black Death, or bubonic plague, which raged through Europe on many occasions but particularly in 1348, killing perhaps a quarter of the total population. This disease is carried by rats and fleas to man, where the organism, *Yersinia pestis*, attacks and enlarges the lymph nodes in armpit, groin and neck, and these enlargements used to be called buboes. Droplet infection from man to man can occur and then the disease may run a rapidly fatal course.

It was obviously vaguely understood that the disease was contagious, for the *Decameron* of Boccaccio started as a result of gentlemen and ladies moving out of Florence to avoid it. In its opening pages the author says, 'No doctor's advice, no medicine could overcome or alleviate the disease' and 'the violence of this disease was such that the sick communicated it to the healthy who came near them, just as a fire catches anything dry or oily near it . . .; and moreover, to touch the clothes or anything else the sick had touched or worn gave the disease to the person touching.' It was about this time that quarantine was introduced, to isolate potential sufferers for 40 days until it was sure that they were not infected. Empirical observation and practice can sometimes be correct, and may have to wait on scientific evidence to validate the reasons for the practice. In this sense science is then an aid to understanding and not necessarily a basis for action. These two aspects of science need recognition.

The undermining of the church's dominant position in the culture of the European Middle Ages came in large extent from an increasingly educated laity, who were able to question the clergy and explore their own ideas independently of dogmatic religion. They did not cast off religion, though they viewed it in a different light from that of conforming clergy. Not all the clergy did conform. Roger Bacon (c.1220–1292) became a Franciscan friar, and he taught and wrote extensively. He is sometimes credited with introducing experimental science, but this has been disputed, though he entertained the idea of experiment, which in itself was unusual. He was a devotee of Aristotle and is said to have been influenced by Avicenna in the Arabian tradition, so that he had a special interest in mathematics, algebra and alchemy, as well as in astrology. He is of interest here as a paradigm of the changing views of the Middle Ages in the recurrences to Greek philosophy, yet modified by other cultural influences that had pervaded Europe. The ground was being slowly prepared for the Renaissance which paved the way for the rise of science and of scientific medicine.

Before moving on to consider the Renaissance it is of interest to consider the state of the art of medicine as the Middle Ages drew to a close. What is sure is that it was only a tiny proportion of the population who had medical care, however indifferent. Physicians in particular were scholars and therefore to be found only in the major centres where intellectual life flourished. Surgeons, the craftsmen, were more widespread because there were more of them, of a sort, and they were so often in attendance on the armies, based on every feudal castle and lord. Fighting was an integral part of the period. Surgeons then knew about the surgery of trauma: treatment of fractures by splinting; reduction of joint dislocations; applying the red-hot cautery to wounds to stop bleeding (this also induced infection, giving rise to the so-called 'laudable pus' which was thought erroneously to be a good sign of healing); applying bandages and salves of various, usually obnoxious, substances; and amputating limbs. They might know of the pain-killing properties of opium, mandragora and alcohol. In cold surgery the more expert surgeon could trephine the skull and remove pieces of the cranium and he could repair hernias in the groin and cut through the perineum to remove stones from the bladder. There were also operations to be performed on the eyes, including one for cataract in which the lens was pushed down with a needle inserted into the eyeball. The thought of all these done without real anaesthesia is enough to induce a shudder now.

Physicians had a slightly lofty approach to their subject. A few diseases had been characterized, but the essence of the profession was to consider symptoms, inspect the patient and his various excreta and then pronounce on prognosis and treatment. This last always involved some alteration of diet, often given in great detail (a habit persisting late into the twentieth century); advice on rest, sleep and exercise; baths and bathing, either hot or cold; and drugs which were usually compounds of so-called 'simples' which were single herbs, roots, leaves and fruits. Looked at from the present-day pharmacology they were nearly all useless, though many patients must have suffered from the administration of emetics, purgatives and expectorants. Not a few must have died of water and salt depletion occasioned by these 'remedies'. It is especially to be noted that physicians did not normally make any physical examination of the patient, so that they could know very little about most internal diseases of heart, lungs, liver and gastrointestinal tract.

Women in childbirth had no medical help. It would have been deemed immodest and sinful for a man to be present at a birth, though apparently some physicians would advise on what to do in cases of difficulty without actually seeing the patient. Also women were very definitely second-class citizens in the eyes of the church and of society, so would scarcely command interest from men at this period of history. The maxim was 'in sorrow shalt thou bring forth' and this is not a recipe for helpful intervention.

There was, of course, no antenatal care, so it was the terrors of labour that occupied the midwives, who were untrained (*Figures 5.3 and 5.4*). They must have had useless nostrums to administer to the parturient women to stimulate her to get on with a prolonged labour. And they would press and knead the abdomen in attempts to force the baby out. It is sure that they must have dragged on the feet and legs of any fetus presenting by the breech. They must have tugged on the cord too to pull out the placenta (afterbirth). They would have been powerless to stem haemorrhage and to resuscitate a baby except by slapping it and perhaps making matters worse. And fits (eclampsia) must have seemed a supernatural visitation and a harbinger of death. Children too were not of interest to the medical profession at this time. They just lived or died, and were subjected to a variety of home remedies when they were ill, while their mothers were showered with advice from old wives.

The scientific background of medicine was virtually non-existent. The prime science is that of anatomy, and this was learned mainly from the butcher's shop, animal dissection and a few human ones. Probably it did not matter much since the state of medicine and surgery could scarcely have taken advantage of any advanced anatomical knowledge. In physiology there was some understanding of the functions of the spinal nerves and presumably of the lungs and gut, but is was at a very rudimentary level and most of the physiological notions were plainly wrong, being based in speculation only. Pathology too suffered because it was still on the wrong lines. It was based in the four humours—white bile, black bile, blood and phlegm—each underlying a particular temperament (bilious, melancholic, sanguine

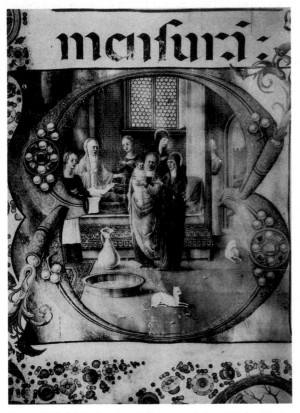

Figure 5.3 A birth-chamber. Miniature, from a MS, by Girolamo da Cremona. (Reproduced by courtesy of the Wellcome Institute Library, London)

and phlegmatic) and these spilled over into the clinical notions of all disease being characterized under the four headings of hot, cold, moist and dry. Of course the treatments were based on these and hot conditions were cooled, moist ones dried and so on. Thus all the remedies available had to be classified under the same scheme. And there remained the notion of plethora, a theory that attributed disease to parts of the body being overstuffed with blood. It is this that led to the remedy of bleeding the patient. This blood-letting, based on a totally erroneous idea, went on for centuries, and must have weakened and killed, directly or indirectly, many thousands of people, all with the best of intentions!

It seems strange now that so little progress had been achieved in just over 2000 years since the days of Hippocrates, but there was no appropriate theory nor technology for it to be otherwise. Yet from here on the pace quickened, slowly at first, as the ideas began to change, and then more and more rapidly, right into the twentieth century. No wonder that this change was and is called the Renaissance as new ways of thinking about the world developed. But the old ways were still there and many of them still remain, and especially to be remembered are the non-specific, non-scientific values of nursing, tenderness, compassion and concern for each sick and dying person, whoever he or she may be. These are constants in the history of medicine which must not be overlooked in the wonders of modern

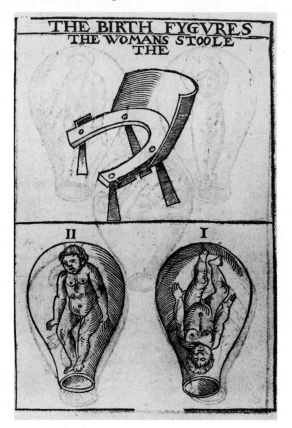

Figure 5.4 E. Roesslin, *The byrth of Man-kynde,* 1540. (Reproduced by courtesy of the Wellcome Institute Library, London)

technology and science. Those virtues and the practices that stem from them owe much, but not everything, to religious forces of many kinds. These too still have their place in the practice of medicine, even though it is not as overt as it once was; but that is true of many activities apart from medicine.

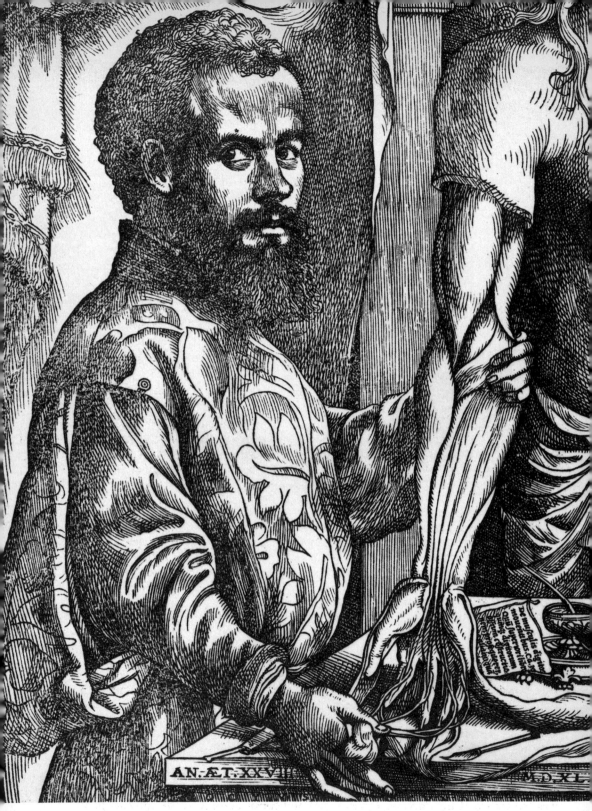

AN·ÆT·XXVII

M·D·XL

Andreas Vesalius [1514–1564] (Reproduced by courtesy of the Wellcome Institute Library, London)

Chapter 6

Renaissance

It is possible to be bogged down in questions of whether there was a Renaissance, and if so what its characteristics were. Historians have modified their views over the past four centuries. But to modern historians there is a discernible pattern of change occurring around the fifteenth and sixteenth centuries which marks a difference from the previous 1000 years or so. In far too stark simplicity it represents a growing independence of the laity from the church and the clergy, and a willingness to consider aspects of the world and human life that had not interested the church in its religion and philosophy. This movement was by no means anti-Christian and anti-Church, for the laity leading it were Christian. They were called Humanists, but they were Christian Humanists. They moved out of the church's spheres of special interest into other ones, concerning Man and Nature. This was done by an appeal and reversion to classical antiquity and a study of the pre-Christian Greek writers and philosophers in particular.

Presumably this seemed innocuous enough at first to the church because it could hardly then have foreseen where this might lead in undermining its authority. Attempts to defend this authority were, however, made and they continue to this day. But the church's authority had already been diminished in its struggles with secular powers and princes, while universities had forged ahead with their studies in law and the humanities and science, largely independent of the church and clergy. No longer were the clerics the nearly sole repositories of learning and of knowledge. It is in this that they were being challenged, though not in any adversarial sense. Whereas the clergy had, almost by default, arrogated to themselves exclusive rights to all knowledge, they were now being shown that there were certain spheres in which their total remit did not run. As a result there could be thought, observation, and later experiment, unconstrained by dogmatic theology. Interpretations of phenomena could be made without consideration of their implications for religion. This change is indeed worthy of a name to mark it and Renaissance is a good one. It seems to signify the origins of the modern world as we know and contemplate it. There was a change in intensity of exploration of the natural world, including Man, and carried on often outside the confines of the church.

What had to be thrown off were many myths concerning Nature. They included the notion that all matter was made up of earth, air, fire and water; that the earth was the centre of the universe (geocentric) and consisted only of the continents of

Europe, Asia and Africa; that planetary motion was circular; that Man consisted of the four humours having the four qualities of hot, moist, cold and dry; and that celestial bodies and spirits in Nature affected the lives of men and women. Getting rid of all these and many more has required immense intellectual effort. Aiding and abetting these changes at the time were geographical exploration and navigation; practical arts and crafts, demanding new technologies, in architecture, building and engineering; and above all the invention of printing with moveable metal type, attributed mainly to Gutenberg in Germany in the mid-fifteenth century. This one technique, and its later developments, may be said to have changed the nature of the human world, in gradually allowing masses of people and not just élites to acquire knowledge, and therefore power. It has forged communities of intellect, which have changed the world and its works, as well as its thinking, by facilitating communication and storing knowledge.

In medicine the community of intellect was perhaps slower to develop than in many other subjects, particularly those of astronomy and physics. Medicine at first did not have suitable technologies available as they were to others, and in many ways it is far more difficult to practise than they are. Medicine is not only a discipline concerned with physical and biological material, but also has psychological, social, cultural, philosophical and religious overtones, often of greater intensity than those affecting what have become known as the natural sciences. They have their cultural connotations but of a different kind than those of medicine.

A milestone for medicine was 1543. In that year Andreas Vesalius (1514–1564) published his *De Humani Corporis Fabrica* (*On the Fabric of the Human Body*) (*Figure 6.1*) while he was at the University of Padua. This was the first anatomical work based on dissections made by the author and produced on the new printing presses. The illustrations were made by Jan Stephan van Calcar, a pupil of Titian (*Figure 6.2*). Both Vesalius and Calcar were Belgians, the first being born in Brussels of a family of generations of apothecaries. He met Calcar in Venice, after he had been a student at the Universities of Louvain and later of Paris. He was always keen on anatomy and dissected many small mammals as a boy as well as animals and human cadavers in Paris. Inevitably he must have been drawn to Padua which was then in the forefront of the teaching of anatomy. Soon he was lecturer in surgery there and in 1537 Professor of Surgery and Anatomy. He went from the University of Padua to supervise the illustrations of his book which were being prepared in Venice, and all was published in Basel, in Switzerland, in seven books. He took the finished work to the Emperor Charles V, who was in Mainz. Promptly he was made physician to the Emperor, and that was the post he had always coveted, for his father had been apothecary to Charles. Because his ambition had been achieved he made no further contributions to the sciences of medicine. He remained in the service of the Emperor and of his son, Philip II of Spain, where he worked in Madrid. In 1564 he made a pilgrimage to Jerusalem, and perished in a shipwreck in the Gulf of Corinth on his way back.

It is a surprising life story. He took the old traditions of Galen and refuted them for Man, saying they were applicable only to animals. He must have been aware of the anatomical work of Mundinus (1316) at Bologna and that of Leonardo (fifteenth century), but he pulled all the previous work together and added to it by careful personal observation and depiction. In so doing, of course, he indirectly called into question much of the received knowledge of physiology of the time. And yet he seems to have done this work almost as a sideline so that he could impress

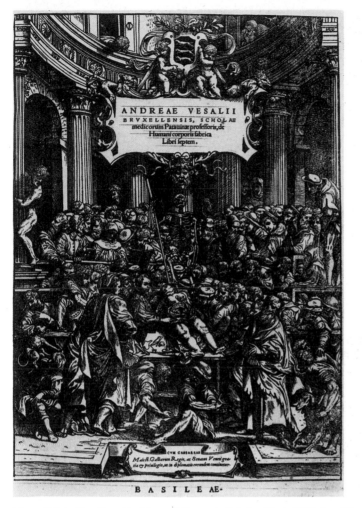

Figure 6.1 A. Vesalius, *De Humani Corporis Fabrica*, Basle 1543, t.p. (Reproduced by courtesy of the Wellcome Institute Library, London)

the Emperor and work for him. Whatever the motives for the work, however, he started new approaches to anatomy and physiology and so began the science of medicine and surgery, as distinct from their practice, and gave a fillip to the study of biology and anthropology. Seldom can a single work have been so seminal, and it was all done before Vesalius was 29 years old.

In the same year of 1543 Copernicus published his *De Revolutionibus Orbium Coelestium* (*On the Revolutions of the Celestial Spheres*), which discarded the notion of Ptolemy that the universe centred round the earth. He substituted the sun as its centre (heliocentric). This too was seminal in re-orientating man's view of the world and his place in it. Moreover, it began new ideas in physics and on the nature of matter. Copernicus was Polish and spent some years in the University of Padua, around 1501, where he studied law and medicine, the prime faculties of the university. He returned to Poland in 1503 and finally settled in Frauenburg where

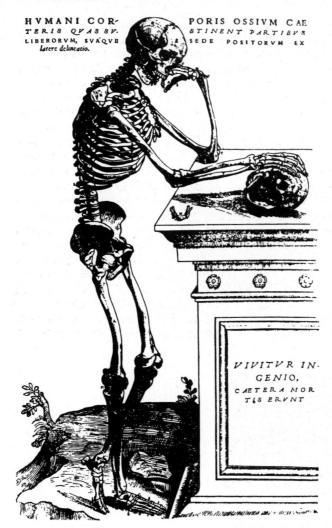

HVMANI COR-
TERIS QVAS SV.
LIBERORVM, SVAQVE
Latere delineatio.

PORIS OSSIVM CAE
STINENT PARTIBVS
SEDE POSITORVM EX

VIVITVR IN·
GENIO,
CÆTERA MOR
TIS ERVNT

Figure 6.2 Skeleton from the anatomical work of Vesalius, 1543. (From *A Short History of Medicine*, 1928, reproduced by permission of Oxford University Press)

he was a representative of the cathedral chapter and a canon. This one year is an incredible landmark for astronomy, physics, biology, anatomy, physiology, medicine and surgery emanating mainly from two men exemplifying the climate of opinion of their age. The change in physics came about since if the sun is the centre of the universe then why objects fall to the ground (gravity) needs explanation, for prior to this it was maintained that bodies naturally fall to the centre of the universe, which in the new theory had changed so that they should fall towards the sun. The heliocentric theory was rapidly accepted in England at the time, and this must later have helped Newton in his formulations about gravity.

   It may seem strange to include here considerations of natural sciences apparently remote from the practice of medicine, but in the final analysis medicine is very dependent on the world views and technologies generated in the basic natural sciences. The presuppositions of natural knowledge are common to all sciences and practices, so that ideas arising within them have some significance for the others, sometimes expanding and developing them, and sometimes limiting their progress.

About this time there was a naming of the anatomical parts, so that the subject was becoming one of public agreed knowledge, at least to the cognoscenti. Vesalius' teacher in Paris, Jacques Dubois (1478–1555), also known as Sylvius (though not he of the cerebral fissure), had named many blood vessels and muscles, though his nomenclature was not published until 1556. It is an impish thought that Vesalius' haste to publish before his former master may have been occasioned, as it often still is, by the wish to be the first in the field. Quickly after his masterpiece came *De re anatomica* of Realdo Colombo (1515?–1559) in 1559. He had worked at Padua before leaving for Rome. Gabriele Falloppio (1523–1562) (*Figure 6.3*), Fallopius, was a student of Vesalius at Padua and followed him as Professor of Anatomy. He is best remembered for discovering the tube running from ovary to uterus and which is now named after him. But he made many other discoveries of cranial nerves and is said to have named the vagina and placenta, though Aristotle is also credited with these terms, meaning 'sheath' and 'cake' respectively. Fallopius had a famous pupil in Fabricius ab Acquapendente, who taught Harvey about the valves in veins. In Rome was Eustachius (1524–1574), who in 1552 published anatomical tables. He is remembered by having given his name to the tube running from the middle ear to the nasopharynx. It is somewhat surprising to find the interest in the ear, for it is a most difficult area to dissect satisfactorily.

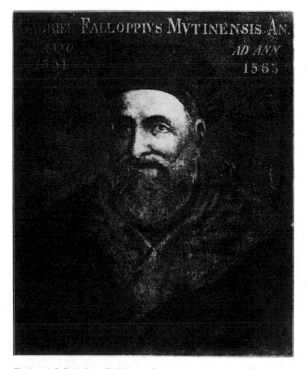

Figure 6.3 Gabriele Falloppio [1523–1562]. (Reproduced by courtesy of the Wellcome Institute Library, London)

It was not a sinecure to be an anatomist then, for Miguel Servede (1509–1553), Servetus, was burned at the stake by Calvin's actions against him because of his book, *Restitutio Christianismi* of 1553. The book was also burned. He is credited with saying that blood passed from the lungs to the heart. Many other anatomists pressed on with the good work during the decades after Vesalius, so demonstrating that when an innovator has shown the way in thought and technology (in this instance by dissection, observation, description and depiction) there are many who follow who will exploit them to the full and so glean an immense amount of additional knowledge, though without the touch of genius of the originators. The process is the one by which science has progressed and still continues to do so.

The basic science of medicine was also on the move. In medicine, as physic, one of the key figures was Paracelsus (1493–1541) (*Figure 6.4*). He was Swiss and rejoiced in the name of Aureolus Theophrastus Bombastus von Hohenheim. He seems not to have been very loveable and to have been impressed by his third name. (He may have given the word 'bombastic' to literature.) He toured Europe gathering information of all kinds, especially medical lore from anyone. He gained a reputation for treatment wherever he went. At Basel in 1527 he became Professor of Medicine and started out by publicly burning the works of Galen and Avicenna, while upholding the works of Hippocrates, and no doubt those of himself. His interest for us is that he seems to have been able to discard the old traditional ways

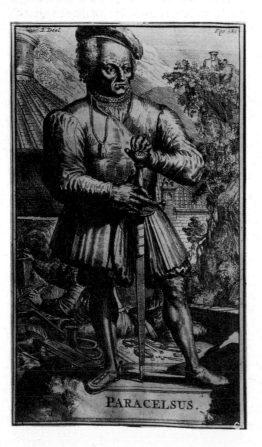

Figure 6.4 Aureolus Theophrastus Bombastus von Hohenheim Paracelsus [1493–1541]. (Reproduced by courtesy of the Wellcome Institute Library, London)

and trust himself and his own observations. Also he grasped something of the importance of chemistry. This was in no fit state to be properly imported into medical therapeutics and understanding, yet this is what he seemed to want to do. In this he was long before his time, but this insight was overlaid and mixed up with a mélange of superstition, folklore, magic and various supernatural spirits. Nevertheless he was, for his time, a fine practising physician and surgeon, and by being so he was able vociferously to oppose many of the more stupid notions of the early sixteenth century, such as diagnosis by looking at the urine or the stars, and advertise the dangers to the public deriving from the attentions of itinerant ignorant surgeons. There is a definite and valuable place for the iconoclast, in preparing the ground for others.

Paracelsus' father taught chemistry, particularly to miners of Augsburg, in southern Austria. No doubt it was this that stimulated the son's interest in things alchemical. He introduced various substances into his practice and pharmacopoeia including laudanum from opium, arsenic, copper sulphate, iron, lead, mercury, potassium sulphate and sulphur. There were, of course, many stranger concoctions. But he carefully described the clinical manifestations of syphilis and prescribed mercury in graduated dosage. He also recognized cretinism and goitre as being allied in some way. In 1536 he published his *Die Grosse Wunderartzney*, a treatise in surgery, in which he opposed meddlesome interference with wound healing, preferring nature to achieve what she might. So he was a massive contributor to his time, and had great influence. He must have been larger than life, with the sparks flying off him in a hotch-potch of muddled ideas, facts and experience, with sometimes astonishing insights and foresight in a miasmic haze of the magic and supernatural. In character, he even perished outrageously in a tavern brawl! It would have been an experience to know him.

Thomas Linacre (1460–1524) (*Figure 6.5*) was a great English physician who ministered to both Henry VII and Henry VIII. He graduated MD from both Padua and Oxford, so he was definitely a child of the Renaissance. This is made certain by the fact that among his patients were Erasmus and More, and also Cardinal Wolsey. Linacre persuaded Henry VIII to found the College of Physicians of London (1518), and he was its first president. The object was to safeguard the status of physicians in and around London and incidentally warn off other practitioners, though much later the College came to be more concerned with standards of medical practice. There were too many mountebanks practising in all sorts of ways at the time, and Linacre's intention was that the College should be the licensing and examining body for physicianly practitioners in London, and the regulation continued for many centuries. This foundation, after Salerno, paved the way for all subsequent endeavours to improve the quality of medical practitioners so that the public shall be best served, by allowing patients to be able to distinguish between practitioners who are properly qualified and those who are not. This initiative is still being worked out in various specialties in the twentieth century. Linacre was a scholar who translated Galen's works from their original Greek, and 4 years before his death he was ordained as a priest in the Roman Catholic church.

Another English physician of note at the time was John Caius (1510–1573) who was a Fellow of Gonville Hall at Cambridge and later this became Gonville and Caius College (1557). He studied in Padua and is said to have shared lodgings there with Vesalius. He was a scholarly physician who wrote on many subjects, and was physician to Henry VIII, Edward VI, Mary Tudor and Elizabeth I. He followed Linacre as President of the new Royal College of Physicians.

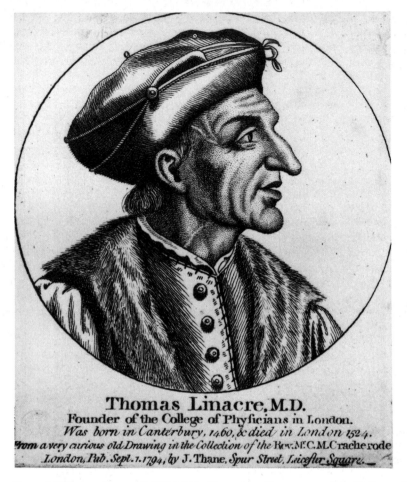

Thomas Linacre, M.D.
Founder of the College of Physicians in London.
Was born in Canterbury, 1460, & died in London 1524.
from a very curious old Drawing in the Collection of the Rev. M. C. M. Cracherode
London, Pub. Sept. 1. 1794, by J. Thane, Spur Street, Leicester Square.

Figure 6.5 Thomas Linacre [1460?–1524]. (Reproduced by courtesy of the Wellcome Institute Library, London)

Some credence might be given to the story that syphilis was acquired by Christopher Columbus' sailors in their voyages of discovery in the New World, which began in 1492. By 1495 there arose in Naples a more acute form of syphilis than is known today, and it rapidly spread throughout much of Europe. It was called the Neapolitan disease at first, but then the French called it the English disease, and the English the French disease, and it was also known as the Spanish disease. Over succeeding centuries syphilis has slowly changed its character from being moderately acute to being very chronic and afflicting the patient over several years, at least until recently when specific remedies have been found to cure the disease. This apparent adaptation of the population to infectious diseases is not uncommon. Tuberculosis similarly was originally an acute disease which became chronic. In isolated communities the introduction of measles, for instance, may decimate the child populace, but over some years the children acquire at least a relative resistance to it. Syphilis came to be so called because of a poem written by Hieronymus Fracastorius (1483–1553) and published in 1530. The title was *Syphilis, sive morbus Gallicus* (*Syphilis or the Gallic Disease*) (*Figure 6.6*). Syphilis was the name of the shepherd who contracted the disease. The signs are described in verse in a very good clinical description. It also gives the treatment by mercury and guiacum, and the first of these drugs was used right into the twentieth century.

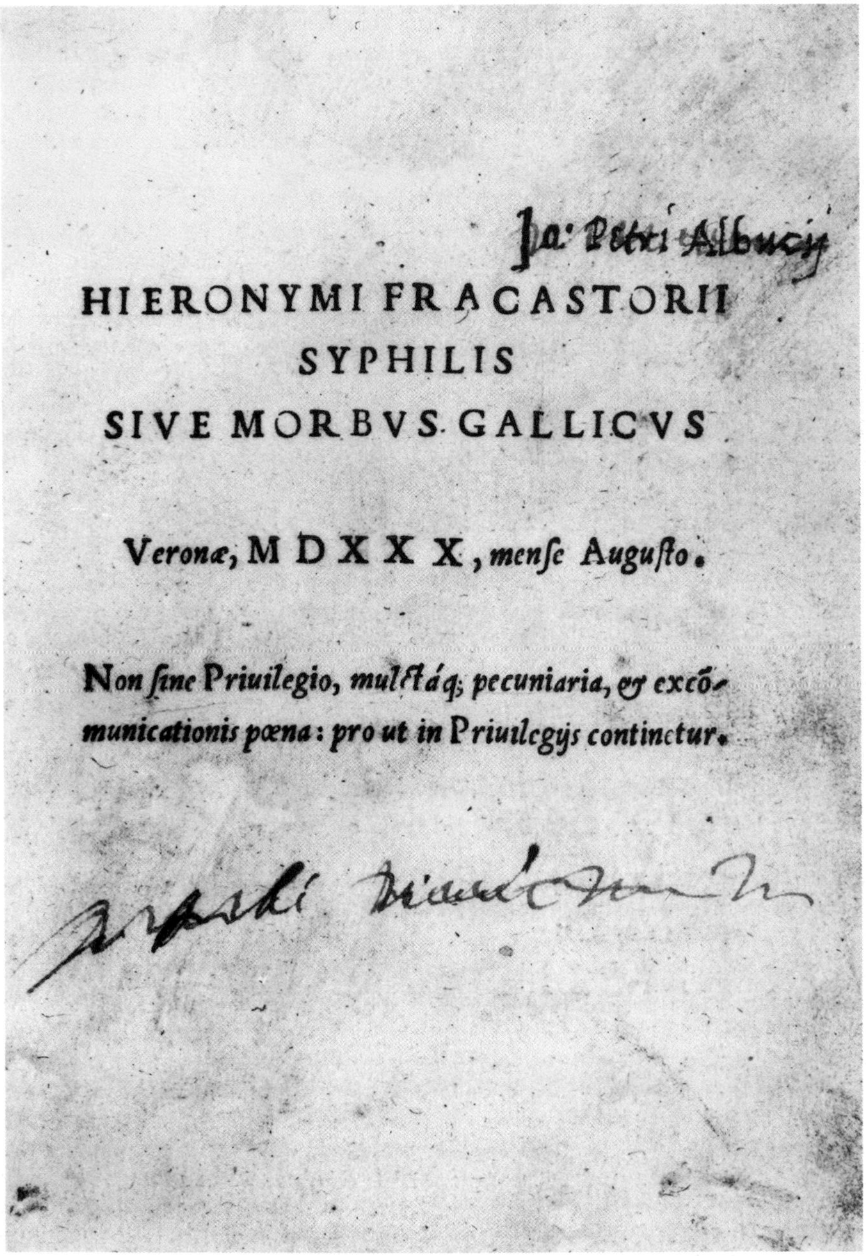

HIERONYMI FRACASTORII
SYPHILIS
SIVE MORBVS GALLICVS

Veronæ, MDXXX, menſe Auguſto.

Non ſine Priuilegio, mulctáq; pecuniaria, & excõmunicationis pœna: pro ut in Priuilegijs continetur.

Figure 6.6 Hieronymus Fracastorius, *Syphilis*, Verona 1530, title page. (Reproduced by courtesy of the Wellcome Institute Library, London)

Fracastorius worked mainly in Verona, where he was born, and he was a contemporary and friend of Copernicus at Padua. From this beginning Fracastorius went on to study other infectious diseases and described the various routes of infection in his *De contagione* of 1546. He even appeared to guess at the possibility of very small particles being the method of transmission.

Guillaume de Baillou (1538–1616), a Frenchman and medical graduate of Paris, recognized and described whooping cough, and first named the disease of rheumatism, differentiating it from gout, though this had been done by Hippocrates. Baillou also revived the notion of the importance of local climatic factors in fostering and helping to start epidemics. He was physician to the Dauphin, thus having connections with a royal court as so many of the famous physicians did.

Caius also described the 'sweating sickness', in a book of 1552. Its nature in modern terms is still unknown, but it raged through England in 1551 in a severe epidemic, which affected whole populations of whom many died. Perhaps it may have been of the nature of epidemic influenza, such as ravaged Europe in 1919.

These examples show the interest in infectious diseases and the first attempts to categorize and recognize them clinically. This is an essential forerunner for further understanding them so that they may be controlled. At first this could only be by such means as isolation of cases and avoidance of contact of the healthy with the sick, so far as that was possible. Without some delineation of clinical characteristics of infections the science of bacteriology could scarcely have begun, as it did in the late nineteenth century. In observing and recording the natural history of various infections the pioneers rendered an invaluable service.

Outshining these important physicians was, however, the French surgeon, Ambroise Paré (1510–1590) (*Figure 6.7*), who deserves to rank with Vesalius for his medical contributions. He ranks too with John Hunter in the development of surgery. He was the son of a cabinet maker in a rustic area and became an apprentice barber in Paris about 1533. That trade was bound up with surgery then and he studied at the Hôtel Dieu, where he learned anatomy and surgery. By 1537 he was an army surgeon, and now is perhaps the most famous of them all. In 1552 he became surgeon to King Henry II and served the three subsequent monarchs too. This is now unimportant compared with the advances he made in practice. Until his time wounds sustained in battle had been treated with hot oil and cautery. The story has it that on one occasion he ran out of oil and had no cautery and so treated wounds with an ointment of egg yolk, rose oil and turpentine. To his surprise the wounds healed better and more quickly with this than with the then accepted methods. A further humane treatment that he introduced was that of ligature of vessels at amputation of limbs. These too had been previously treated with hot oil or pitch and the red-hot cautery to stem the bleeding. By this gentler treatment he must have saved hundreds from agonies beyond description.

He avoided operation when he could and in herniotomy he preserved the testis rather than sacrificing it as so many surgeons did. This was, of course, the re-introduction of old methods which had been described but not widely adopted. But his fame and reputation brought them to the attention of lesser practitioners. He struggled for the welfare of his patients by introducing artificial teeth, and eyes and limbs, with all of which he was forever experimenting. Of course the materials and technology were crude by present standards but were marvels for their time. And another aid was that of the truss for hernia, showing a real will not to subject his patients to surgery that might be avoided.

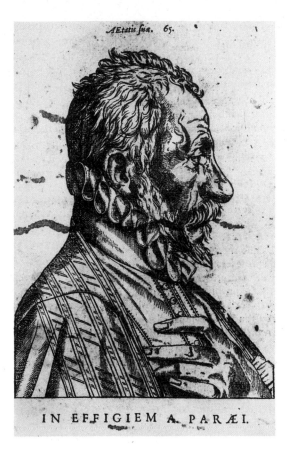

Figure 6.7 Ambroise Paré. (Reproduced by courtesy of the Wellcome Institute Library, London)

Paré's famous saying was '*Je le pansait; Dieu le guarit*', ('I dressed him; God healed him'), which is a fine statement of the creed of the surgeon in aiding and not frustrating the *vis medicatrix naturae*. He failed, however, to cure King Henry II who was wounded by a lance in a tournament. The weapon penetrated the head just above the right eye. Vesalius was sent for from Brussels and together these two dissected four heads to try to decide what the lance might have injured. This must have been one of the earliest recourses to the laboratory to solve a pressing clinical problem.

He made a major contribution to obstetrics too in re-introducing internal version, in which with a hand passed through the vagina and cervix in difficult labour the fetus is turned round so that the presenting head is pushed up out of the pelvis and a leg brought down and outside the woman's body, where it can be pulled on to extract the baby. Although relatively dangerous both to mother and child this operation can be lifesaving when labour is obstructed with no chance of delivery by any other means. The result of prolonged obstruction is certain death for both mother and baby. At least internal version offered a chance of life to both, in the days when both caesarean section and forceps could not be used, since the latter had not been invented and the former was a death sentence for the woman. However, Paré did err in perpetuating the notion that during labour the pelvic bones separate to a reasonable degree. This suggests that by waiting sufficiently long delivery will be possible by natural means and without interference. Not even the very great can be right always, and this was a great man of outstanding humanity, curiosity and humility. Some have staked a claim for him as the 'father of surgery', and such an epitaph would be justified.

Paré wrote treatises on gunshot wounds (1545), on internal version (1550), and on surgery (1564). In this last he described fracture of the neck of the femur, pain on micturition due to enlarged prostate gland, and suggested that syphilis was a cause of aneurysm, which it is. He wrote too of those helpful adjuvants such as massage and exercise and especially nursing care.

He nearly came to a tragic end at the hands of the mob at the massacre of St. Bartholomew's Day in 1572, for he was suspected of being a Huguenot. He was sheltered by King Charles IX and so escaped. In fact he was twice married under Roman Catholic rites and his children were baptized in that church. Perhaps the suspicion arose because 2 days before St. Bartholomew's Day he had attended the assassinated Admiral Coligny, the Huguenot general. It was this murder, with others, that sparked off the massacre.

Meantime, in this sixteenth century, midwifery was not standing still. Women in childbirth had been relatively neglected for centuries by the medical profession because of cultural constraints. There was, of course, no antenatal care, which is a product of the twentieth century. There was not much medical help either in the tribulations and difficulties of labour. Women in these parlous straits could only call on ignorant midwives and unskilled relatives and friends. Yet in 1500 a Swiss sow-gelder, Jacob Nüfer, had performed a successful caesarean section on his own wife, when doctors had given her up for lost. Presumably from his trade he had just sufficient knowledge of anatomy and the tools to do the job. Both mother and baby survived and she lived to produce several other children, all of which is near incredible considering the odds stacked against the whole family.

Eucharius Rösslin (died 1526) was elected city physician for Frankfurt-am-Main in 1506. Somewhere about 1450 the town had received a legacy which was to be used for the provision of midwives to the poor women of Frankfurt. This is probably the first example of some form of governmental control of the practice of midwives. Rösslin produced a book for them in 1513 quaintly called *Der Schwangern Frawen und Hebammen Rosengarten* (*The Rose-garden for Pregnant Women and Midwives*) (*Figure 6.8*). He acknowledges a debt to many of the older writers on midwifery, but especially his book is derived from Moschion (*fl.* sixth century AD) who took most of his material from Soranus of Ephesus (*fl.* second century AD). Moschion had written in Latin for Roman midwives and in question and answer form. Rösslin, of course, was writing also in the local vernacular. By 1532 his son, also called Eucharius, had translated *The Rose-garden* into Latin as *De Partu Hominis*, and later editions included pictures taken from Vesalius. In England the book was translated into English by Richard Jonas and published by Thomas Raynalde. By then it had become known as Raynalde's *Byrth of Mankynde* (1540). It was dedicated to Katherine Howard, wife of Henry VIII. It held the field as the main textbook of midwifery until the last edition in 1676. From this it can be gleaned that very little new or scientific was imported into midwifery practice, which must have remained virtually stagnant for more than 1500 years. Yet at least interest was awakening in the problems of labour and attitudes to women were probably slowly changing too. They might have been very definitely second-class citizens, but even this is better than being of no account at all.

Other German cities introduced municipal midwives, and towards the end of the

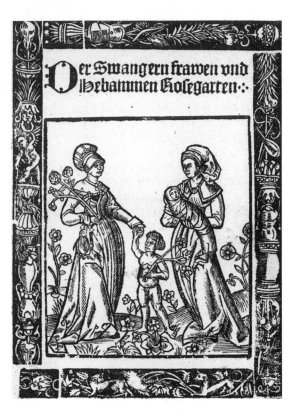

Figure 6.8 Eucharius Rösslin, *Der Schwangern Frawen und Hebammen Rosengarten*, Hagenau 1513, title page. (Reproduced by courtesy of the Wellcome Institute Library, London)

century in 1596 there appeared Scipione Mercurio's *La Commare o Riccoglitrice*, which described the operation of caesarean section, and what had become known as Walcher's position in which the legs of a labouring woman are extended over the end of the bed so that the extreme extension of the hips shall enlarge the bony pelvis as much as possible, so helping to overcome obstruction, when the baby's head is too large or the pelvis too small (known as disproportion). It is now of little use. Perhaps the re-introduction of internal version by Paré was the single most important advance in midwifery in this century, though there were recorded 15 successful cases of caesarean section. Following close behind this in importance for the future was the investigation of the properties of ergot by the physicians of Marburg in Germany (1596). They showed how it could be used to make the uterus contract in labour and after it.

Despite these advances in midwifery it has, however, to be recorded that in 1591 Agnes Sampson in Edinburgh was burned at the stake for attempting to relieve the pains of labour. The clerical writ in the subjection of women still held sway despite a few enlightenments. Yet the church was under siege from within as well as from without, since Luther in 1517 began the Reformation, by criticizing abuses within the church, so establishing Protestantism, which was later to develop in many forms.

Although they were only straws in the wind there were incipient moves to improve the public health. Stews (brothels) in Southwark were suppressed in 1506. In 1532 bills of mortality were published by parishes in London. In 1538 Henry VIII ordered the keeping of records of christenings, marriages and deaths. Apothecaries were legalized under an Act of 1543, so that there were regulatory bodies for them as well as the physicians and barber–surgeons, at least in London. Elsewhere in Europe the regulation of midwives is not to be forgotten either. The search for the maintenance of standards for the health care professions is therefore no new phenomenon. In 1593 there was an Act against overcrowding in dwellings in London and 5 years later the first Poor Laws were enacted making each parish responsible for the relief of the indigent.

The scientific background too was changing. Exploration and navigation needed astronomy. There had been the voyages of Amerigo Vespucci and of Christopher Columbus. From 1519 Magellan voyaged round the world. Drake did the same in 1580, and scurvy (lack of vitamin C) afflicted his crews.

In 1568 Mercator produced his maps, which because they took into account the rendering of the round world in two dimensions were more accurate than any previous ones.

The nature of the physical world began to be understood in a quite different way from previously by the works of Giordano Bruno (1548–1600), Tycho Brahe (1546–1601), Galileo (1564–1642), and Johannes Kepler (1571–1630). Bruno extended the concepts of Copernicus by suggesting that the universe was infinite. For his pains he was burned at the stake as a heretic, but he had furthered the diminution of Man in the scale of things. Brahe was a careful collector of observations about the heavenly bodies, devoting his life mainly to this. In 1572 he saw and plotted the course of a new star, which on previous theory should not have been there. The result was an upholding of the Copernican idea of a heliocentric universe. Brahe realized that the planets revolved round the sun, but thought that the whole system revolved round the earth. He did this remarkable work without the benefit of the telescope. Kepler was fortunate in having a professor at Tübingen who believed in the Copernican cosmos and it was on this that he built. His first work *Cosmographic Mystery* (1596) he sent to Brahe, whose observatory he joined near Prague in 1600. When Brahe died a year later Kepler had full access to all his records, which he analysed further. The result was that he enunciated laws of planetary motion, showing first that Mars had an elliptical orbit round the sun, and not a circular one. This completely upset the mediaeval notion of celestial spheres moving in perfect circular orbits. Moreover, he showed a mathematical relationship between the distance of a planet from the sun and the time required to complete its path around the sun. This was obviously paving the way for Newton.

Kepler also began the study of optics by suggesting that luminous bodies gave off light in every direction but that a cone of light reached the eye and was then focussed by the lens on to the retina. He realized that if the resultant point of light fell in front of or behind the retina then vision would be blurred. He was thus able to explain why spectacles were valuable for those with poor eyesight, for this had been a mystery before. He widened his observations by tracing the paths of light in the telescope which had recently been invented, probably by Galileo.

By the end of this century the philosophy of the Middle Ages had begun to be overturned. The world of nature was being opened up and subjected to detailed observation and even sometimes experiment to verify hypotheses. Observation was aided by optical instruments, the telescope and microscope. Lenses were of course known and simple magnifying glasses had been used for a long time. But in 1590 Hans Jansen and his son Zacharias in the Netherlands introduced the compound microscope in which two or more lenses are combined to produce larger images of small objects. Very quickly this was applied to the observation of insects and other living things, even though the objects were crudely prepared and the lenses of poor quality compared with later times. This preparatory work and new ways of thinking led to the remarkable discoveries of the seventeenth century associated with Harvey, Francis Bacon, Descartes, Boyle and above all Isaac Newton.

By the end of this remarkable century anatomy was established. At first it had comparatively little impact on the practice of surgery, which was empirical rather than scientific. It did, however, provide a basis for the study of function in physiology as in hearing (Eustachius) and optics (Kepler). There came appreciation too of bones, joints, muscles and the distinctions of nerves from tendons, and of arteries from veins. Chemistry was being touched on by such as Paracelsus. Medicine was in a descriptive phase, which was essential to all future progress, and much of its concern was with infectious diseases, the great killers for centuries. Surgery was gentler and more humane in the hands of Paré. Obstetrics at least made a start by reviewing what was known from antiquity, though social factors probably prevented it from moving forward very much. There were glimmerings of a concern with public health. Apothecaries, barber–surgeons, physicians and midwives came sporadically under some sort of control of their practices in which they had to have some entry qualifications to their professions, some experience in practice and to be examined. All was rudimentary, but showed the way for future development. And the natural sciences of astronomy and of physics, with optical technology, were changing the concepts of the physical world.

SIR ISAAC NEWTON

DRAWN AND SCRAPED MDCCLX BY IAMES MACARDEL FROM AN ORIGINAL PORTRAIT
PAINTED BY ENOCH SEEMAN NOW IN THE POSSESSION OF THOMAS HOLLIS F.R. AND A.SS

ES ITALIENS CES PEVPLES INGÉNIEVX ONT CRAINT DE PENSER LES FRANÇA
ONT OSÉ PENSER QVÀ DEMIE ET LES ANGLAIS QVI ONT VOLÉ IVSQV'AV CIEL *PAR*
V'ON NE LEVR A POINT COVPÉ LES AILES SONT DEVENVS LES PRÉCEPTEVRS D
ATIONS NOVS LEVR DEVONS TOVT DEPVIS LES LOIX PRIMITIVES DE LA GRAVIT
ION DEPVIS LE CALCVL DE L'INFINI ET LA CONNAISSANCE PRÉCISE DE LA I
IÈRE SI VAINEMENT COMBATTVES IVSQV'À LA NOVVELLE CHARVE ET À L'I

Sir Isaac Newton. (Reproduce by courtesy of the Wellcome Institute Library, London)

Chapter 7

Newton's century (Seventeenth)

The year 1600 saw Giordano Bruno burned at the stake for believing the universe to be infinite; Fabricius ab Acquapendente published his work on the valves of the veins; and William Gilbert (1544–1603) published *De Magnete* (*On Magnetism*) (*Figure 7.1*). Bruno paved the way for Galileo, Kepler and Newton; Fabricius for Harvey; and Gilbert, with many others, for Newton.

Gilbert was a physician, appointed to Queen Elizabeth I in 1601 and at her death in 1603 to her successor James I of England. He followed Copernicus in believing the world to be heliocentric, but in being among the first to study magnetism he was investigating a force acting over a distance and invisible. He knew that magnets pointed north and south on the earth's surface, that the northern end of the needle tilted towards the earth, and he concluded that the earth acts like a bar magnet. He thought that the planets were held together by a force of magnetism, and the parallel with gravity is close. He also investigated electricity, such as it was then, and first used terms such as electric attraction, force and magnetic pole. It might be thought that all this has little to do with the history of medicine, but it has already been emphasized how medicine is quite dependent on prevalent world views. Gilbert was helping to change these, and it is now commonplace that many human corporeal phenomena are of an electrical and magnetic nature. Electrophysiological technology now is of great importance in diagnosis and treatment. Without some such pioneers as Gilbert, none of this would have been possible.

Kepler (1571–1630) was busy with optics (*see* previous chapter) and by 1609 Galileo (1564–1642) was using both the telescope and compound microscope, both of which he improved. Technology was thus enlarging the range of observation, making it more accurate and detailed, so inevitably reacting on and modifying theory and philosophy.

Francis Bacon (1561–1626), an influential man of his day, appointed Lord Chancellor of England in 1618 and Viscount St. Albans in 1621, published his *Advancement of Learning* in 1605. His importance for the present theme is not what he actually deduced about science and knowledge, but rather that he was groping for an understanding of them and their methods. In this it is to be assumed that he was representing something of the concerns of his time. Though by no means the first in the field he drew attention to the method of induction which builds up firm instances of phenomena and then draws general conclusions from them. From this philosophical position onwards he began to make mistakes as

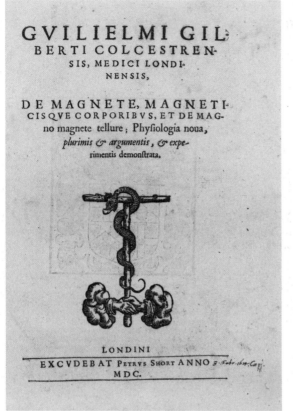

GVILIELMI GIL·
BERTI COLCESTREN-
SIS, MEDICI LONDI-
NENSIS,

DE MAGNETE, MAGNETI-
CISQVE CORPORIBVS, ET DE MAG-
no magnete tellure; Physiologia noua,
plurimis & argumentis, & expe-
rimentis demonstrata.

LONDINI
EXCVDEBAT Petrvs Short ANNO ꜣ·ꜰₑᵦᵣ·₁₆₁₄·Cₒᵣⱼ.
MDC.

Figure 7.1 Title page of Gilbert's *De Magnete*, London 1600. (Reproduced by courtesy of the Wellcome Institute Library, London)

judged by present beliefs, but his general notion of induction has had its value in the development of scientific thought. He struggled with the sorts of relationships that might exist between nature and the mind of man, which demand at least some unspoken beliefs, if not rational thought, for science to develop.

Galileo (1564–1642) (*Figure 7.2*) was primarily a mathematician, and he is quoted as saying that 'The Book of Nature is written in mathematical characters', a belief now embedded in the philosophy of science, either for good or ill. It is at least possible that this restricts the fields of science too greatly. After initial life at Pisa he became professor of mathematics at Padua. He defined the motion of pendula and showed that bodies of different weights fall to the ground with the same acceleration. Before his time it was believed that heavier bodies fell faster than lighter ones. Unfortunately it seems to be myth that he did this work from the top of the leaning tower of Pisa.

His astronomical observations through the telescope showed a new star where only 'fixed' stars should have been. In Greek times the Aristotelian notion was that the heavens, at least in the far distance, were unchanging and perfect. Galileo upset this idea, and this is important for it heralds the importation of change into natural phenomena—a change from the static to the dynamic world view. Biological process depends heavily on change. Living beings are not fixed. If they were, evolution and process would not be possible. This commencing idea, brought into

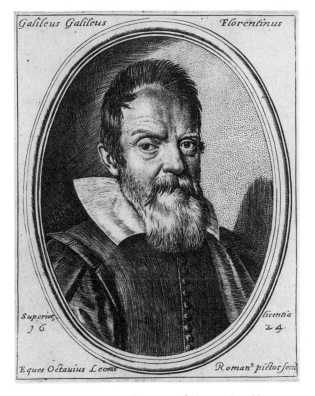

Figure 7.2 Galileo Galilei [1564–1642]. (Reproduced by courtesy of the Wellcome Institute Library, London)

the scheme of things by Galileo, can be seen to be a forerunner of present-day biology and medicine. It is interesting that the church, and the scholastics within it, had some inklings of the dangers for them and their doctrines of this change in thought, for Galileo was indicted by the Inquisition and had to make a half-hearted declaration that the new Copernican system for the universe was wrong and the Ptolemaic system right, since it accorded with the scriptures.

Protestantism too was advancing and loosening the monopoly of knowledge of the church and the scholastics. The change must have been particularly galling for them, for in the words of Basil Willey, who took St. Thomas Aquinas as the paradigm of the scholastics, 'Galileo typifies the direction of modern interests, not in refuting St. Thomas, but in taking no notice of him.' This really is a profound change in the direction of thought, liberalizing it and virtually licensing men to investigate what they will without prior permission from clerical and scholastic authority. It was in escaping such authority that the Pilgrim Fathers set sail for New England in 1620, and further Protestant emigrations took place later. This rebellion went very far when Charles I was executed in 1649 and Cromwell took over the Commonwealth until 1660. This brief incursion into general history shows that the movements in science and in medicine were not isolated phenomena in refuting the old scholasticism and church authority.

René Descartes (1596–1650) (*Figure 7.3*) was a mathematician and philosopher, helping unwittingly to overthrow scholasticism and to set the scene for science, and

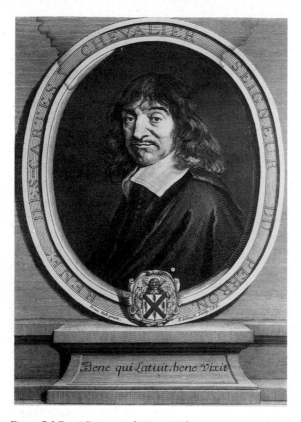

Figure 7.3 René Descartes [1596–1650]. (Reproduced by courtesy of the Wellcome Institute Library, London)

much of medicine. His famous dictum '*Cogito ergo sum*' (I think therefore I am) was a succinct statement separating mind from matter. Galileo had done this too in saying, 'I do not believe that there exists anything in external bodies for exciting tastes, smells and sounds, etc., except size, shape, quantity and motion. If ears, tongues, and noses were removed, I am of opinion that shape, quantity, and motion would remain, but there would be an end of smells, tastes and sounds. . . .' The importance of these two statements is that they firmly recognize a physical world 'out there' distinct from human beings which is amenable to the exercise of observation and experiment and mathematics, and that because of his mind man can, as it were, separate himself from that physical, natural world.

This has immense implications for deciding on the nature of Man and his relationships with the world outside him, but this must wait for later discussion. The obvious separation of mind from matter has had repercussions on the development of psychology, psychiatry and sociology, which in some eyes have made them quasi-sciences. This Dualism, as it has been called, may or may not have been detrimental to these subjects.

Further than this, however, Descartes had the vision of a grand design of a universal science. This could be no more than intuition at the time, but its later fruits have shown that there really is a continuity between physics, chemistry, biology and all their associated phenomena. This has allowed interpretation of some sciences in terms of those of another, usually in forms of reductionism of biology to chemistry and chemistry to physics, rather than construction of greater complexity from the simpler elements. Because of his vision Descartes wrote his *Discourse on Method*, published in 1637. It was in elegant French, when the usual vehicle would have been Latin. Almost incidentally to its theme it formulated optical laws of refraction, explained the rainbow and introduced co-ordinate geometry. The method, in order, consists of (i) doubts and the clearing of the mind, (ii) analysis of the problem to be solved, (iii) collecting evidence from the simpler to the more complex instances, and (iv) checking the reasoning of the argument. In the book he managed to deny the presence of mind to all creatures except Man, so that the rest of biological creation had to be purely mechanical. It can be seen that this concept may lead to many difficulties in some spheres, but opens the way to the investigation of biological mechanisms in physicochemical terms.

That path has been very productive, though it has led to problems in the latter half of the twentieth century. As so often with new concepts there are those who push them to extremes, and so arose a school of iatrophysicists who wished to interpret everything medical in physical terms. Later, with the rise of chemistry, came the iatrochemical school, who put everything down to chemistry. Later still came Georg Ernst Stahl (1660–1734) who discarded both physics, chemistry and even anatomy as bases for medicine and imported a concept of animalism and vitalism imbuing the biological and human worlds with special forces which could not be demonstrated in terms of other sciences. He was professor of medicine at Halle. None of these schools added anything of value to medical progress, though they generated many futile arguments sustained with some heat. Each school may contain the germ of a little truth which is elevated to a great one. The process still goes on now, with sects over-emphasizing diet, exercise, psychology, herbs, meditation, vegetarianism, alternative medicine and so on. All these movements have their truths, which are not so all-consuming as their devotees would have others believe. And it is only fair to note that the same is true of orthodox medicine and science too.

In chemistry the paradigm of the century was Robert Boyle (1672–1691), who published *The Sceptical Chemist* in 1661. This finally disposed of the Aristotelian elements of earth, air, fire and water and of the three principles of mercury, sulphur and salt invoked by Paracelsus. Boyle demonstrated his law that at a constant temperature the volume of a gas is inversely proportional to the pressure applied to it. He postulated that chemical actions occur between particles which are in motion, so providing a theoretical atomic basis for subsequent work, and accepting the change of the world view from static to dynamic. He was particularly fortunate in his assistant Robert Hooke (1635–1703), who demonstrated his law that the elasticity of solids is dependent on the force applied to them. He published studies in astronomy and in microsocopy, being the first to name the cell from the cavities seen in a specimen of cork (*Micrographia*, 1665). He showed that animals in a vessel from which the air was evacuated died, and that an animal with an open chest could be kept alive by artificial respiration, brought about by a bellows in the trachea. He was a superb experimentalist and demonstrated many of his works to the new Royal Society, which was granted a royal charter in 1663.

The Royal Society of London for the Improvement of Natural Knowledge had its beginnings a few years before 1663, in some informal meetings of scientists, who persuaded Charles II of their importance. The first roll of fellows is of almost incredible virtuosity, including many doctors, as well as Boyle, Hooke and Christopher Wren, and later were Samuel Pepys and Isaac Newton, both of whom became president. Fellows have retained pre-eminence through the succeeding three centuries by their contributions to science (natural knowledge). The significance of the society's founding lies in the revolution in thought that it publicly marks. Among the most illustrious of early Fellows was Newton (1642–1727).

Newton is the founder of modern physics. He made significant contributions in optics, mechanics, astronomy and mathematics. He formulated the law of gravity as a universal force. He analysed light into its spectral constituents, and believed it to be corpuscular in nature. His three laws of motion are not in detail relevant here, nor is the law of gravity, except in so far as they exemplify the completeness of the change that had been wrought in the thinking about the way in which nature works, and how it might be investigated and how general laws about its behaviour may be deduced. The masterly book epitomizing this is the *Principia Mathematica* (*Philosophiae Naturalis Principia Mathematica* or *Mathematical Principles of Natural Philosophy*), published in 1687 by the Royal Society. Almost incidentally to help him with his work he invented the infinitesimal calculus, though this discovery he shared with Leibniz (1646–1716), who also communicated papers to the Royal Society. His philosophy conceived of the world as made up of monads or separate particles.

This exegesis of him and of Newton is, of course, far too compressed and simple, but the purpose is only to show the groping after a universal system of nature, governed by universal laws moving from the simplest particles of uniform kind yet combining to give the richness and complexity of the world as seen by Man. This is in fact the view now vindicated by all subsequent scientific work. The sequence of increasing complexity runs from subatomic particles to atoms, to molecules, to physics and chemistry, and on to biochemistry and biophysics, through to cells, organs, living entities, to Man and his psychology and sociology. All at base is essentially simple, but by combination and recombination of elementary substances the complexity of the world emerges. And this mode of thought has its origins mainly in Newton's century. He is its exemplar by drawing together so many strands of his age. Yet Newton was an avowed Christian. He recognized two books, the Bible and Nature. This simple statement embodies a profound change in attitude from earlier times.

In the sciences more directly basic to medicine we have to return to the early years of the century. Sanctorius of Padua (1561–1636) invented a clinical thermometer, though this was not used in clinical medicine till much later. Using a modified form of pendulum he was also able to count the pulse and this too was forgotten in practice. But he is remembered as a founding father of physiology and of the investigation of metabolism. By continuously weighing himself in a specially constructed balance he showed the effects of eating a meal and showed that 'invisible perspiration' occurred through the loss of water from the skin and lungs, without sweating (*Figure 7.4*). The eminence of Padua was still being maintained by him and also by Fabricius ab Acquapendente (1523–1562). It was in 1600 that he wrote on the valves of the veins. Perhaps he did not realize their significance in full, though he was a great teacher.

William Harvey (1578–1657) (*Figure 7.5*) studied in Padua, after graduating from Cambridge, for about two and a half years around 1600. It was he who appreciated the function of the venous valves and those of the heart in allowing the flow of blood in only one direction. The thought had occurred to many that the old ideas of

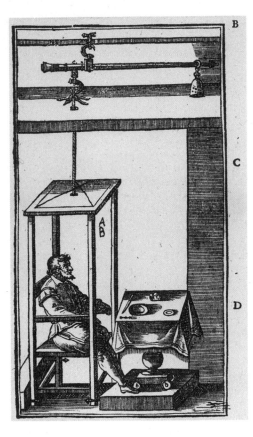

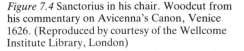

Figure 7.4 Sanctorius in his chair. Woodcut from his commentary on Avicenna's Canon, Venice 1626. (Reproduced by courtesy of the Wellcome Institute Library, London)

oscillation of the blood and the doctrine of the pneuma and vital spirits were becoming less tenable. Some had even suggested the possibility of a pulmonary circulation (e.g. Colombo of Padua). Presumably Harvey picked up some of these notions, though he still revered Aristotle and Galen on his return to London in 1602. Here he ultimately became physician to St. Bartholomew's Hospital and to King Charles I, whom he accompanied in the Civil War. He was a learned physician and active in the affairs of the Royal College of Physicians. His treatments were conservative, and it is strange to think that his ideas of the circulation of the blood had comparatively little influence on his practice. The practical use of his experimental and observational work had to wait till much later. This is not unusual, for pure science is not always rapidly converted to applied science. That has to depend on further technological advance.

Harvey practised and dissected many varieties of animals and in 1616 he gave a series of lectures at the Royal College of Physicians, essentially on anatomy. It seems that he then adumbrated the idea of the circulation of the blood, and the work was finally published in his *De Motu Cordis et Sanguinis in Animalibus* (*On the Motion of the Heart and Blood in Animals*) in 1628 (*Figure 7.6*). He demonstrated that the flow of blood in the veins was always towards the heart, by the simple experiment of placing a finger over a full vein, stroking the vein towards the base of the limb to empty it as far as the next valve, and then removing the finger to show that the vein filled from the periphery. It was elegant and simple.

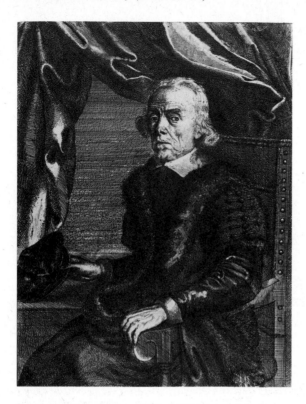

Figure 7.5 William Harvey [1578–1657]. (Reproduced by courtesy of the Wellcome Institute Library, London)

He showed too that the valves of the heart must operate in the same way, and that there were no communications between the right side of the heart and the left. He demonstrated that the systolic contractions of the ventricles expelled the blood in only one direction and that the arteries pulsated because of the shock wave transmitted along their walls from the beating heart. They did not pulsate of their own accord. And he showed how bleeding from cut arteries and veins differed in the two. Because the ventricles are of equal size and blood is not lost it must be that the blood circulates through the lungs and through other parts of the body. This whole demonstration was a superb display of the uses of hypothesis, observation, experimental demonstration and logical deduction, all interrelated and acting on one another to come to a definite and irrefutable conclusion. It is for all these things that Harvey can be looked on as a genius. It remains to be noted that despite this logic he was severely criticized in his day by some of his contemporaries. Perfect scientific logic is by no means always persuasive to those with closed minds steeped in the past, unable to shake off the myths they have learned.

Harvey was also one of the founders of embryology. In 1651 he published his *De Generatione Animalium* (*On the Generation of Animals*). This was not so important as the *De Motu Cordis* though he did maintain that the embryo gradually developed by differentiation and was not entirely preformed in the hen's egg, simply to grow bigger with the passage of time. This is essentially correct and helped to establish

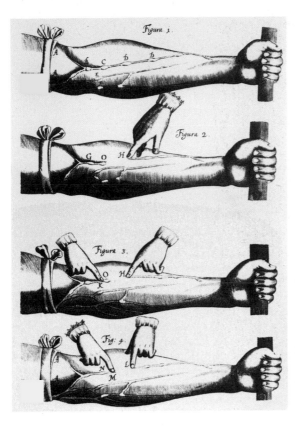

Figure 7.6 Experiments to demonstrate
the function of the valves in the veins [to
keep one-way blood flow], from Harvey's
De Motu Cordis, Frankfurt 1628. (Reproduced by courtesy of the Wellcome Institute Library, London)

epigenesis as against preformation, a doctrine that had been held by many up to
that time. He did not have the benefit of a microscope so it is remarkable that he
advanced as far as he did and even that he had an abiding interest in embryonic
development. This may have been partly derived from his sojourn in Padua, for
Fabricius and others there investigated and wrote on the subject.

Harvey's only lack in the understanding of the circulation was that he could not
see how the blood moved through capillaries in the tissues from the arteries into the
veins. These tiny vessels had to wait for the researches of Marcello Malpighi
(1628–1694) who demonstrated them microscopically in his *De Pulmonibus* (*On the
Lungs*) in 1661 (*Figure 7.7*). He was professor of anatomy at Bologna, Pisa and
Messina, as well as being physician to Pope Innocent XII. His observations
convincingly supported Harvey. Malpighi was also a great embryologist and first
saw the aortic arches, the various folds that the embryo undergoes and the optic
vesicles. He worked too on the microscopy of the viscera and his name is still
eponymously associated with structures in the skin and spleen.

The microscope was a major tool of biological research in this century. As a
compound of two lenses it had been discovered in Holland around 1600 by
Zacharias Jansen and improved and used by Galileo. It was also in Holland that
advances were made by Antony van Leeuwenhoek (1632–1723) of Delft and Jan
Swammerdam (1637–1680) of Amsterdam. Both communicated discoveries to the

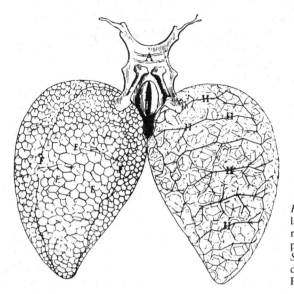

Figure 7.7 Lungs of frog, showing the capillary vessels from a figure by Malpighi in the rare first edition of his work *On the Lungs,* published at Bologna in 1661. (From *A Short History of Medicine,* 1928, reproduced by courtesy of Oxford University Press)

Royal Society and it may have been these that interested Hooke to pursue his own studies. The instruments were very crude. Neither glass nor mechanical nor biological technology were capable of more. Yet the observations made were remarkable. There were no staining methods, yet Leeuwenhoek saw red cells and capillaries, spermatozoa and muscle fibres. Swammerdam produced a *Bible of Nature* (1669) often concerned with insects, and he was also responsible for the muscle–nerve preparation of the frog in which a nerve is left attached to the muscle, so that the nerve can be stimulated by pinching (or electric current nowadays), and the muscle then contracts. Using this he showed that the volume of the muscle does not change during contraction. This observation disposed of the previous notion that something flowed from the nerve to the muscle during contraction. By such comparatively simple observation and experiment may the truth be approached and prejudiced unfounded speculation be swept away. So much of science is devoted to disproof as well as to positive demonstration.

In gross anatomy there was still progress. Thomas Willis (1621–1675) was a professor at Oxford and moved to London to prosecute a successful practice as a physician. His *Cerebri Anatome (Anatomy of the Brain)* of 1664 described not only the brain but also something of its blood supply. His name is still attached to the circlet of vessels at the base of the brain. Francis Glisson (1597–1677) was Regius Professor of Physic at Cambridge, and published his *Anatomia Hepatis (Anatomy of the Liver)* in 1654. The peritoneal capsule of the liver is named after him. Like others of his day he was not a pure anatomist and his clinical observations on infantile rickets were published in *De Rachitide* (1650). Others became interested in lymph glands and lacteals (the lymph vessels which often contain a milky fluid). These glands must often have been enlarged by tuberculous infection at that time. Thomas Wharton wrote about them in 1656. There were dozens of other anatomists too in this century, each adding a mite to the knowledge of anatomy and often adding his name to a structure he had discovered and described. Only the late twentieth century has tended to discard anatomical eponymy, with some loss of colour for the subject.

Some of the anatomical observations were made on cadavers with disease, so that post-mortem pathological observations were perforce made. However, these did not come together as a separate element in the development of medicine until the eighteenth century. It is surprising too that all this intellectual activity had comparatively little impact on the general approaches to clinical medicine. Sir Thomas Browne (1605–1682), the famous literary physician of Norwich, published his delightful *Religio Medici* in 1643. As literature it is a joy, but it shows a mind divided between religion and science, in which the authority of the scriptures nearly always tends to hold the upper hand. It is not a medical treatise, but rather an exposition of the philosophy that guided a physician of the times in his life. An even greater hotch-potch of ideas pervades *The Anatomy of Melancholy* (1621) by Robert Burton, who was not a doctor but a parson. The interest in the book lies in the fact that it roams around many subjects, including medicine, and may show something of the attitudes of enlightened opinion towards the subject. Neither this book nor Browne's shows any appreciation of Harvey's work and the general ferment of biological ideas of the early century. This, with many other historical observations, suggests that we may still be often unaware of the significant movements of ideas around us that may shape the future and we may instead spend our energies on what may turn out to be ephemeral and of no lasting consequence. The thought should be sobering, but probably is not.

Anatomical observations almost inevitably are bound up with the question of the functions of various structures. Some surprising work for the time was therefore done on digestion and respiration, and many other physiological subjects. Regnier de Graaf (1641–1673) of Holland investigated pancreatic juice in 1664. Stensen (1638–1686) worked on salivary and lacrimal glands. Others were concerned with locomotion. In 1669 Richard Lower (1631–1691) of Cornwall showed that dark venous blood passing through the lungs of an animal became bright red, and he concluded that something had been taken up from the air by the blood. In 1665 he essayed the transfusion of blood from one animal to another. John Mayow (1643–1679), like Lower also from Cornwall and Oxford, analysed the movements of respiration and allied these with the uptake of something from the air into the blood. Again there were many others pursuing similar paths to understanding.

In clinical medicine was Thomas Sydenham (1624–1689), often referred to as the English Hippocrates. He studied at Oxford and Montpellier and seems to have been indifferent to the views of his contemporaries. He found little use for the scientific knowledge being garnered around him. In this he was almost certainly right for his time. The knowledge was of small practical value in the treatment of the sick. He therefore redressed the balance as he saw it by reverting to clinical observation at the bedside in the Hippocratic tradition and the Cartesian one of clearing the mind of preconceived notions that could not be tested. His concentration was on what could be done for those who were ill. The scientific contributors laid emphasis perhaps more on understanding. This dilemma of those who are just interested in what they observe and experiment on, and those who want observations and experiments of immediate practical use, is still with us. It emerges in the arguments about pure and applied science, and the place in the hierarchy of esteem of technology. The debate has been sterile for centuries and will remain so. All these branches of knowledge are aspirations of similar nature, reaching out for similar goals, with varying degrees of patience and impatience, which more describes individuals' casts of thought than real differences on the road of what, it is hoped, is progress.

Learning at the bedside has a fluctuating history. It seems to have been used by Hippocrates, but was later largely lost. It was resurrected occasionally, as in Salerno and Padua, but was probably never massively practised. Physicians might listen to the patient and observe him and his secretions and excretions, then fit his illness into some authoritarian theory, such as that of the humours and principles, or those of Galen. In fact Sydenham did subscribe to such theories and yet unwittingly took no notice of them in much of his work. What you think you think may not accord with what you do. He described malaria, gout, scarlet fever, measles, broncopneumonia, pleurisy, dysentery, hysteria and chorea. His famous work of 1683 was on gout. He eschewed many of the complex therapeutic compounds extant in his day, preferring the so-called simples from plants and he used Peruvian bark (quinine) and opiates. He extolled the virtues of fresh air in sick-rooms and of exercise by riding horses. He tried to equate disease with climatic conditions, just as Hippocrates did. His great contribution, however, was not in theory but in the restoration of clinical observation and the description of the natural history of disease as indispensable methods for the progress of medicine.

In surgery there were various treatises, but they do not appear to have shown much progress from the days of Paré. There were bold and clever operators, but again it has to be noted that the advances in scientific thought and philosophy, and those in physics, astronomy, chemistry, anatomy, microscopy and physiology, had no immediate impact on practice. Apparently, all of these needed a period of assimilation and wide diffusion before they could be put to use. Moreover their use had to wait for other technology so that the gap between basic science and clinical medicine could be bridged.

In obstetrics Louise Bourgeois, midwife of Paris and a pupil of Paré's, published a work in 1609. This became *The Compleat Midwife's Practice Enlarged* of 1659 in a London edition. It seems she used Paré's method of inducing labour early in cases where the pelvis was deformed, often because of rickets in childhood. Hendrik van Deventer (1651–1724) of the Hague in Holland wrote also on deformities of the pelvis and their effects in obstructing labour. His interests lay in orthopaedics as well as midwifery. The first English translation of his work came out in 1716 as *The Art of Midwifery Improved*.

Hendrik van Roonhuyze (1622–1672) of Amsterdam in 1661 published a work that described caesarean section, which he may have performed successfully on many occasions, and also describes cases of ruptured ectopic pregnancy and of vesicovaginal fistula, for which he proposed a rational method of repair, to stop the constant dribbling of urine through holes in the bladder opening into the vagina. Such fistulae are commonplace when there is prolonged obstruction in labour and the baby is almost too big to be delivered vaginally. When it is finally delivered it is almost always dead and the vagina and bladder have been grossly damaged. A further major contribution was by François Mauriceau (1637–1709) of Paris. His *Traité des Maladies des Femmes Grosses* (*Treatise on the Illnesses of Pregnant Women*) of 1668 is a classic. He disposed of the prevalent view that the pelvic bones separate during labour, so enlarging the bony birth canal. This wrong belief prevented greater investigation of the problems of obstructed labour, which caused the deaths of countless thousands of women and their babies.

These various works show overtly the state of the art of obstetrics. There was also interest in the early development of the embryo and fetus and the mechanism of fertilization. Because of lack of the appropriate technology and theory these interests did not get very far when judged now. It has been mentioned that there were works by Fabricius and Harvey among others. And it was the Dutchman Regnier de Graaf (1641–1673) who in 1672, from Leyden, published his work on the organs of generation of women. He saw the follicles in the ovaries which are still named after him.

Beneath the surface of the progress of obstetrics in this seventeenth century was, however, the extraordinary story of the development of the forceps (*Figure 7.8*). It is the story of the notorious Chamberlen family. Dr William Chamberlen (?1540–1596) fled the persecution of the Huguenots in France, to Southampton on the south coast of England. He probably had the germ of an idea of making a form of metal tongs, which could be used to grasp the baby's head as it lies low down in the mother's pelvis during late labour. Not uncommonly the head gets stuck there, particularly if the head is large and the pelvis small. There is no room for the hands to reach inside and pull on the slippery head. Others had had similar ideas for many decades, but none of the inventions were of practical use. But William Chamberlen seems to have solved the problem, at least partially. Astonishingly he kept it secret and it was kept in the family and not divulged for about 150 years! Nostrums of many kinds were then kept secret in order to enhance the reputations and incomes of practitioners, so perhaps there was nothing too unusual in this behaviour. William handed on the secret to his sons.

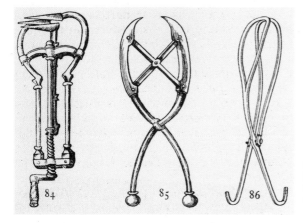

Figure 7.8 Early obstetric instruments. (From *A Short History of Medicine*, 1928, reproduced by permission of Oxford University Press)

The genealogical tree of the Chamberlens is very confusing. There were so many sons and daughters, and the names of Hugh, Paul, John and Peter recur in several generations. The detail is unimportant here, though interesting, and fully dealt with in Walter Radcliffe's excellent little book *The Secret Instrument*. In the story of the obstetric forceps Hugh (1630–?) is of special interest. He practised in London, and when called to a confinement he carried the forceps in an enormous box in order to deceive others as to what it contained. Moreover the metal of the instrument was bound round with leather thongs to prevent the noise of the parts clanking together. It was at that time easy to conceal them in the labour room, since modesty demanded that a sheet covering the parturient woman should sweep over the pudendal region and be tied to the obstetrician's neck, so that he could feel but not see his patient's nether parts.

The cleverness of the Chamberlen forceps was that the two halves of the tongs could be separated at the point at which they crossed over one another. This allowed each blade to be inserted separately into the pelvis to grasp the baby's head and then a pin could be inserted at the cross-over point, allowing the head to be gripped and drawn out of the pelvis. If the cross-over point is fixed it will be understood that the blades have to be separated so far that they cannot be inserted into the pelvis, for the distance between them it too great.

Hugh was a thrusting entrepreneur who was constantly in trouble with the Royal College of Physicians for sharp practices of many kinds. In 1670 he journeyed to Paris to sell the invention of the forceps to Mauriceau. He was given a rachitic dwarf to operate on and not surprisingly was unable to deliver her even with the aid of his forceps. He failed to sell the secret, but he brought home a copy of Mauriceau's book which he translated and so is said to have netted £30 000. He was responsible for many other dubious schemes, and so were the rest of his family. Yet a few of them became court physicians and accoucheurs. The name of accoucheur had been first used for Jules Clément, who attended the Marquise de Montespan when she had a baby by King Louis XIV. It was he who bestowed the title for this service to his mistress.

Hugh's son, also called Hugh (1664–1728) was more orthodox in his education, though he was something of a mountebank too. He went to Emmanuel College, Cambridge and then to Padua and after some problems became a Fellow of the Royal College of Physicians. He had apparently less interest in midwifery than others of his family and from about this time and early in the eighteenth century the forceps gradually became known and used more widely. From this strange and prolonged history came the instrument that transformed the practice of midwifery and has been of incalculable benefit to women and their children. Something of its importance was recognized at the time, for the elder Hugh was elected a Fellow of the Royal Society in 1681, where his contemporaries were Christopher Wren, Pepys, Newton and Boyle.

Beginnings were made in what has come to be called social medicine and epidemiology with the publication in 1662 of Graunt's *Natural and Political Observations upon the Bills of Mortality*. This was an analysis of the causes of death as revealed by the bills, which were collections of data about deaths, and from which indirectly have sprung all vital statistics about populations, as distinct from individuals. In 1683 Dr William Petty followed this with similar analyses, in a book called *Political Arithmetick*. And in 1700 Ramazzini of Modena published *De Morbis Artificium Diatriba* which was the first work on diseases of various trades, of which he described about 40. Occupational medicine of a sort may then be said to have begun.

The seventeenth century marks the beginnings of science and shows the germs of many ideas which have since come to fruition. The rate of change in scientific thinking increased greatly. It is this that has imbued all subsequent progress, by observation, careful recording, experiment and analysis in medicine, as in so many other spheres of human knowledge and practice. Yet science and clinical medicine scarcely came together so that each could react on the other for mutual benefit. There was opposition, often intense, to what we would now accept as obvious and proven, without any hint of doubt. This seems to be an inevitable concomitant of progress, which is compounded of thesis, antithesis and synthesis. There was an admixture of mumbo-jumbo too, as in *Religio Medici*, and shown by the fact that in 1654 Charles II touched about 4000 people in the widely held belief that this would cure them of the King's Evil, or scrofula (tuberculosis). There were several pharmacopoeias too as well as herbals with unsubstantiated claims for the efficacy of drugs and concoctions in various ill-defined illnesses. In English perhaps the most famous has become the *Pharmacopoeia Londinensis* (1649) of Nicholas Culpeper.

A feature of the century was the felt need to disseminate knowledge more widely than previously. This task had been mainly in the hands of the church for many centuries. The invention and use of the printing presses had allowed the publication of more secular works, though books were relatively expensive and in small runs. Universities were founded in some numbers and journals came to be published. Among these were several in Germany and Italy and the *Philosophical Transactions* of the Royal Society started in 1664–5. It is noteworthy too that the centres of learning in medicine spread outwards from Padua and other places in northern Italy to Montpellier, Paris, to Holland in Leyden and Amsterdam particularly, and to London and Oxford.

There was a founding too of professional societies in many countries, all somewhat similar to the Royal Society. And following the founding of the College of Physicians in London in 1518 and the guild of Barber–Surgeons in 1540 came the Royal College of Physicians in Edinburgh in 1681, partly by the influence of Robert Sibbald (1641–1722) and others who had been students at Leyden. There is an interesting story to be written of the progress of medical learning from Italy to Holland to Scotland and onwards to the United States of America. In all these places, in the founding of institutions, it was almost unconsciously becoming recognized that medicine has a public function for the benefit of society as a whole and is not just a simple transaction between one doctor and one patient at a time. There are needs for education, the maintenance of standards of practice, the diffusion of knowledge and skill, and so the protection of the public from the ministrations of the ill-qualified, the totally unqualified and the quacks. These were therefore highly significant moves, in their infancy then but which have grown to be of immense importance now in relationships established between society and medicine.

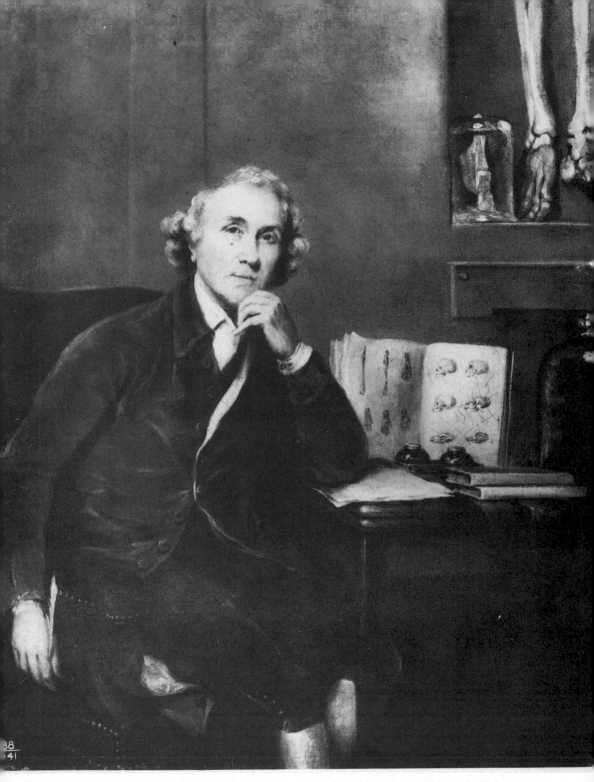

John Hunter [1728–1793] (Reproduced by courtesy of the Wellcome Institute Library, London)

72

Chapter 8
The century of enlightenment (Eighteenth)

In the eighteenth century there are no towering figures in science to compare with Newton in the seventeenth and Darwin in the nineteenth. These two changed the understanding of the world of nature and of Man. The eighteenth century forms a bridge between them. Much was happening, of course, but in a lower key. It is almost as though the intellectual scientific community needed time for rest, recuperation and relaxation after the shock of Newton. It needed time to work on his ideas and to gather more facts and observations on the lines that he had shown to be fruitful. There were many major discoveries and shifts in thought in this century, though they now seem comparatively to be of second order rather than first. The very highest peaks are reached on very few occasions in the history of medicine and science. It is a general truth that after the introduction of new ways of thinking or of new ways of doing by the few, there follows a massive application of the new methods by dozens, by scores and ultimately hundreds and thousands of others. The pebble is dropped into the pool but the ripples spread far and wide in all directions, agitating ever more and more molecules of water. The general process is visible everywhere in medicine today. A new operation (say) is developed by the wit of a small team. The technique and the results are published and disseminated. It is taken up by more and more surgeons, then becomes standard, and finally merits a few paragraphs in a textbook.

It will be remembered that Newton, with many others before him, showed that there is a world of physical nature 'out there' and separable from the mind of the observer. That external world is measurable for it has mass and spatial relationships. (This leads to materialism and mechanism as philosophies.) Measurement and observation can be made almost as if the observer were not part of the process. That physical world exists in its own right and is subject to laws of nature which are everywhere the same. Indirectly these are the laws that God has ordained for matter, so that scientific investigation to look for and establish these laws is a pious occupation and not incompatible with religious views of the world. The external world is quite devoid of qualities that sentient beings impose upon it. It has of itself no colour, no smell, no sounds and no taste. These are put there by the special senses, as Galileo noted.

Despite its apparent simplicity and conformity with modern common sense, once this scientific view of the world is accepted it does pose some difficulties. If the sense organs and mind are adding these qualities to what is observed, then how can that same mind know just what it is observing 'out there' in the material world? The question is still not finally answered, and in this sense science rests on slightly unsure philosophical foundations. It is not therefore surprising that this is the century of Locke, Berkeley and Hume—philosophers to whom the question was important.

John Locke (1632–1704) lived mainly in the seventeenth century, but his influence went into the eighteenth. He was a physician who taught at Oxford, and was medical adviser to the 1st Earl of Shaftesbury, a notable statesman of his day. Locke's interests were in politics and morality and also in natural science. Indeed he collaborated with both Boyle and Sydenham and was a Fellow of the Royal Society at its founding. He was inevitably caught up in the vicissitudes that affected his patron, and it is noteworthy that he had periods in Paris and Montpellier and finally some years as an exile in Holland, all of which were centres of learning and tolerance, and true heirs of the Renaissance spirit. In 1690 he published *An Essay Concerning Human Understanding*. The details of the work are not important here, though in the wrestling with the relationships of the observer to nature they are pertinent to the whole of the later development of science. One feature of his thought was that natural science cannot give complete certainty but can get close to it with careful observation, reasoning, and the application of mathematics where possible.

Bishop George Berkeley (1685–1753) is well known because of later misinterpretation of his philosophical position. This is Idealist, in that it denies material 'out there', believing that knowledge and the bases on which it is built are all in the mind. This is unfair to him and too compressed, but is introduced here to remind of the two extremes of idealism and materialism, each of which, when thoroughgoing, lead to positions that are untenable by common sense. *His Treatise Concerning the Principles of Human Knowledge* was published in 1710.

David Hume (1711–1776) produced *An Enquiry Concerning Human Understanding* in 1758, after many revisions. Again the details are not important here, but the title alone shows the continuing concern about questions raised by the work of Newton. Hume was a sceptical philosopher and showed the inconsistency of beliefs about cause and effect, and he expressed doubt about the method of induction. However, he too returned to the world of common sense whenever he left his study, his books, and writing. He and the other philosophers show how profound a change had been wrought in thinking about the world. Prior to these two centuries it was believed that there were ideas innate in any person which could be reached purely by introspection. After this time there came increasingly the idea that the mind develops from babyhood onwards purely out of the experiences that impinge upon the body and brain. Such ideas still have their effects in the interpretations of psychology, psychiatry and sociology, and the understanding of human mental and social development.

Of course the world of science in the eighteenth century simply ignored these intellectual struggles as irrelevant, just as Galileo had ignored the scholastics. There was work to be done on Newtonian lines in finding out natural laws. This gave rise to attempts at systematization and of the piling up of examples of phenomena, in an inductive method, in the hope that with enough examples a generalization would result. Tyros in experiment even now seem often to cling to the same idea. What is needed instead is an hypothesis about a particular piece of nature which is to be proved or disproved. The thinking and reasoning comes before the collection of appropriate data and not vice versa. But in the eighteenth century collection and systematization was important and reached fruition in Carl von Linné (1707–1778), more usually known as Linnaeus. He was a Swedish physician, interested in botany. He classified plants, animals and minerals in his *Systema Naturae* (*System of Nature*) of 1735, though there were many later editions. This introduced the form of classification still used of giving each organism two names, one denoting the genus and the second the species, as in *Homo sapiens*.

This clearly must have had an influence on biological thought leading up to Darwin, though Linnaeus believed that each species was fixed for all time with no possibility of change over the years. The notion of constant change had not been learned, despite its demonstration in astronomy several decades earlier. The compartmental walls between branches of knowledge are hard to break down. The significance of generalizations in one sphere are not recognized in another.

Another valuable beginning was made by Linnaeus in his *Genera Morborum* (*Types of Diseases*) in 1763. It was then realized that despite the immense variety of presentations of illness in individuals, there were recurring characteristics of disease that enabled them to be grouped together for recognition. This can lead to concepts of diseases that seem to have an identity of their own in isolation from the people in whom they occur. This presently irks many who believe that this view ignores the whole person, making medical practice unfeeling and remote. They wish instead to see whole-person or holistic medicine. This is laudable, but in the eighteenth century the separate identification of diseases was essential to progress. Some pattern had to be extracted from the chaos of disease to make medicine possible at all. There were many others also concerned with systematization in a variety of subjects. One was Johann Friedrich Blumenbach (1752–1840) of Göttingen, who started off craniology and anthropology in his *On the Native Varieties of the Human Race* (1776).

The passion for systematization and the search for universal laws extended to medicine in the schools of iatrophysics, iatrochemistry and animalism and vitalism, as mentioned in the previous chapter. The adherents of these schools hoped to interpret all disease and its treatment in terms of mechanism, or chemistry, or some special quality of biological material. Benjamin Rush (1745–1813) of Pennsylvania went so far as to attribute all disease to a single cause. Despite this aberration he was perhaps the most eminent physician of his day in the United States. In the last quarter of the twentieth century there are still sporadic attempts by individual authors to reduce medicine to a system of law with general applicability. None has so far received acceptance, but they show how strongly people wish to reduce chaos to order, and ultimately simplicity.

Science and medicine, however, are still not yet at that stage. Order and pattern emerging from the welter of natural phenomena can only be achieved in discrete areas of knowledge. The massive general patterns, such as those of gravity or evolution, await some further genius who sees correlations between things, where they have not been seen before. Yet these two laws show that speculation on the grand scale is just as important for the progress of science as the gathering of facts and observations, as well as experiment. The grand hypothesis is important for the generation of the littler ones. And at first both Newton's and Darwin's laws were very large, almost speculative, generalizations built on a small number of special instances.

In physics the matters of importance for medicine were the invention of various thermometers by Fahrenheit (1709) by Réaumur (1731) and by Celsius (1742). However, none of these immediately entered into the practice of medicine at that time. In 1753 Benjamin Franklin (1696–1790) of Boston, USA, installed a lightning conductor, brought in bifocal lenses for spectacle wearers, and treated paralysis with electricity. In 1792 Luigi Galvani (1737–1798) of Padua published his work *De viribus electricitatis in motu muscularis* (*On Electrical Powers in the Movement of Muscles*). He had suspended frogs' legs by copper wire from an iron balcony railing. As the feet swung and touched the iron uprights the legs twitched, because of an electrical potential difference between iron and copper (*Figure 8.1*). Alessandro Volta (1745–1827) of Pavia followed this and showed that muscle can be made to contract tetanically by the passage of an electric current. This was written up in his *Letters on Animal Electricity* of 1792. He also produced the famous Voltaic pile, which was essentially the first electric battery. These works showed that biological phenomena are associated with electrical changes. Ultimately this has had immense consequences in medicine and biology.

In chemistry Joseph Black (1728–1799), a Scotsman, destroyed the theory that held that when a substance burns it gives off a substance called phlogiston. This should entail loss of weight in the residue, but Black showed that in fact it gains weight; so something had been taken up from the air and not lost to it. He came very close to identifying oxygen and he also recognized that when quicklime is heated a gas (carbon dioxide) is given off, and that this is normally present in air. These observations all came out about 1757 and were followed in 1766 by Cavendish who discovered hydrogen, and by Rutherford who discovered nitrogen in 1772.

In that year Joseph Priestley (1733–1804) isolated oxygen, but his notions about it were confused and he spoke to the Frenchman Antoine-Laurent Lavoisier

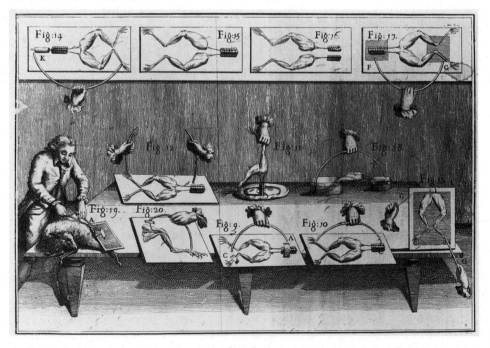

Figure 8.1 From A. Galvani, *De viribus electricitatis*, Modena 1792. (Reproduced by courtesy of the Wellcome Institute Library, London)

(1743–1794), who quickly understood its place in the scheme of things. Lavoisier recognized oxygen as important in respiration and compared this function with combustion, a view that has stood the test of time. Like others before and after him he did not get all the way to full understanding, but he took a long step in the right direction. To complete these eighteenth-century investigations of gases of medical interest came Sir Humphry Davy (1778–1829) (of miner's lamp fame) with the discovery of laughing gas (nitrous oxide) in 1799. Despite all this activity in chemistry and in physics, the discoveries still had no real impact on clinical medicine. They led to some further understanding of physiological processes but there was no way in which they could yet be imported into practice.

In anatomy, then still the main scientific basis of medicine, the torch of learning was slowly transferring from Padua to Leyden in Holland. One of its famous professors was Franciscus Sylvius (1614–1672) who preserved the study of anatomy at a high level. Hermann Boerhaave (1668–1738) (of whom more later) was the inspiration of Leyden medical education over many years. Bernhard Siegfried Albinus (1697–1770) was his pupil and professor of anatomy and surgery at Leyden in 1718 and subsequently moved to the chair of medicine in 1745. Albinus and Boerhaave caused the works of Vesalius to be edited and re-published, and in other books based on the system of that master, Albinus used excellent artists. This interest in medicine, and its scientific basis in anatomy, slowly moved to Edinburgh. Several students from there studied at Leyden. Sibbald has already been noted as a founding father of the Royal College of Physicians of Edinburgh in 1681. Another was Archibald Pitcairne (1652–1713), who became a professor of medicine appointed by the town of Edinburgh in 1685 and for 1 year he was professor of medicine in Leyden (1692). He was there a teacher of Boerhaave. Out of his energies and those of the Monros sprang the world-renowned Edinburgh Medical School.

John Monro (?–1737) was a student of Pitcairne's, and it was he who started the school. He specially instructed his son Alexander (1697–1767) so that he should become professor of anatomy at Edinburgh, which he duly was at the age of 22. There were still problems in anatomical dissection in those days, and this Alexander Primus had to escape the mob when he was accused of body-snatching from graves or prior to interment. In 1758 Alexander was succeeded in the chair of anatomy by his son, Alexander Secundus (1733–1817). He held the appointment for 50 years and it is his name that is attached to the foramina in the brain. In 1798 the chair passed to his son, Alexander Tertius (1773–1859), and he held the professorship for a further 38 years. Unfortunately he returned to the practice of simply reading out lecture notes which had belonged to his grandfather(!) so he made no great contribution. As in the previous century there were dozens of advances, based on gross dissection, made all over Europe. Many names were attached to bodily structures. But the best general treatise of anatomy was published by Samuel Thomas Soemmerring (1755–1830) from Frankfurt in 1791–6 with the title *Vom Baue des menschlichen Körpers* (*On the Anatomy of the Human Body*). He had made excellent researches on the cranial nerves, and on the ear, nose and throat. The book remained in vogue for over half a century.

In physiology the Reverend Stephen Hales (1677–1761) of Teddington in Middlesex first measured the blood pressure (1733) by inserting a goose's trachea (for flexibility) into the carotid artery of a horse. The trachea was attached to a glass tube and he was able to see how far up the tube the column of blood was carried, and he measured the height. He also introduced the concept of artificial ventilation of the lungs. It was a time when all educated gentlemen could indulge their fancies of dabbling in science, but few did it with such good effect as Hales. In another sphere the clergyman Gilbert White (1720–1793) published his *Natural History of Selborne* (1789). Though nothing to do with medicine, its spirit of careful recording, observation and depiction were in keeping with the age and its methods.

The giant of physiology was Albrecht von Haller (1708–1777). He came from Bern in Switzerland, studied in Leyden, but moved to the newly founded university of Göttingen, as professor. Like so many others of his time he was a polymath, making contributions to anatomy, to physiology and medicine and the arts, for he wrote poems and novels. He carried out hundreds of experiments and distinguished the excitability of muscle from the sensitivity of nervous tissue (1757). Between 1759 and 1766 he published his monumental *Elementa physiologiae corporis humani* (*Elements of the Physiology of the Human Body*). Slowly the science of physiology was emerging, to be enlarged later.

A further science basic to medical practice is pathology. By post-mortem investigation it shows the changes brought about in the body by disease. The end-result of a morbid process is displayed, and from this it may often be possible to infer what went wrong in function, and how. Moreover it gives insight into the causes of the living patient's symptoms and signs. With the upsurge in anatomy previously outlined, it is surprising that these truths were not earlier recognized. It remained for Giovanni Battista Morgagni (1682–1771) to begin the study of morbid anatomy which he did by tireless investigation, when he was professor of anatomy at Padua. In his *De Sedibus et Causis Morborum* (*On the Sites and Causes of Disease*) of 1761 he published his results in about 700 cases, correlating what he found *post mortem* with the clinical picture in life. Here was anatomy for the first time being actively used in the progress of medicine as practised clinically. Of course it had always been of some value in the practice of the simple surgery of those years, but since surgery was so limited in what it could be used to do, much of anatomy was of little value to the surgeon. The continuing eminence of Padua is noteworthy. Two sciences basic to medicine—anatomy and pathology—began here, and both are still extensively used in practice.

Morgagni was interested only in naked-eye appearances. François Xavier Bichat (1771–1802) of Paris, however, used the microscope to begin to define the histological changes produced in tissues by disease. His work *Traité des Membranes* (*Treatise on Membranes*) was published in 1800. Prior to this, in 1793, Matthew Baillie (1761–1823), a Scot practising in London, published *Morbid Anatomy*. It was well illustrated and depicted the emphysema of the lungs of Dr Sam Johnson, the outstanding literary figure of the metropolis. It is now impossible to conceive how medicine could be practised and understood without gross and microscopic anatomy of the dead. And of course this has been extended into diagnosis in the living by biopsy of organs, in which a piece of tissue is removed and then examined in a variety of ways, including histology, in the laboratory. By the end of the eighteenth century therefore there were the beginnings of understanding not only of normal structures and functions, but also of abnormal structure and function. It was a tremendous step forward, not fully appreciated at the time.

Clinical examination of the patient was very different in the seventeenth and eighteenth centuries from what it is now. Little, if any, distinction was made between symptoms and signs. Now symptoms have come to mean the subjective description of what the patient feels and tells to the doctor. Signs are the 'objective' things about the patient elicited by the doctor, using the methods of inspection, palpation, percussion and auscultation. In these two centuries signs were virtually never elicited. Instead the doctor listened to the recital of symptoms, looked at the face but often no other parts of the body, and inspected the urine, sputum and pus or other excretions and secretions (not faeces), then pronounced a diagnosis and treatment. This often led to consultation by letter and the issue of a prescription, without the patient being seen. Today telephone consultations and instructions on treatment are deeply frowned upon! All the appropriate evidence on which to base a diagnosis has not then been obtained, and this may constitute negligence.

The dominant physician of the eighteenth century was Hermann Boerhaave of Leyden. He was a master of languages, classics and mathematics. He was appointed as a teacher in the university in 1701 and gave lectures on anatomy. In 1709 he was professor of botany and medicine and by 1718 he was professor of chemistry. All the while he practised as the most sought-after physician of his day. His enormous contribution was as a teacher and inspirer of his students, many of them taking what they had learned from and through him to all parts of Europe and especially to Edinburgh. He published *Institutiones medicae* (1708), *Aphorismi* (1709), *Index Plantarum* (1709), and *Elementa Chemiae* (1731) showing his mastery of medicine, botany and chemistry and his ability to profit from the posts he held and to disseminate to others what he had learned. In some ways he was a great man rather than a scientist, and some of his writings have been criticized by historians. Yet towering personalities have their place in the progress of medicine as well as the lesser ones. They stimulate and inspire others to achieve more than they might have done in different circumstances. Unconsciously, perhaps, they perceive the needs of their times and understand them, so handing them on to their pupils and successors. It may be through them that great teachers may ultimately be known for their achievement.

Although Boerhaave has here been taken as the exemplar of medicine, it has to be remembered that the degree of specialization that we accept now was not present then. So the Monros of Edinburgh were physicians too, as were many others of those previously mentioned. A pupil of Monro Primus was William Cullen (1712–1790), who held chairs of medicine and chemistry both in Edinburgh and in Glasgow, the latter of which he helped to found as a medical school in 1744. He too was a fine teacher, lecturing in English rather than Latin—the usual custom then.

Clinical investigation began to improve in this century. A few physicians measured the temperatures of their patients. But most significant was the work of Leopold Auenbrugger (1722–1809) of Vienna on percussion. He reported this in his *Inventum Novum* (*New Invention*) of 1761. Like all new methods it was not widely accepted at first, though now it is an essential part of medical investigation, particularly in diseases of the chest. Auenbrugger noted the sounds elicited from various parts of the body and in a variety of pathological lesions, such as fluid-filled cysts, when one finger is used to strike another on the surface of the body. From these observations he tried to deduce the nature of structures deep inside the body cavities. An important side-effect of this method was that it meant the skin had to be exposed and the doctor had to touch the body as well as inspect it, so that general clinical examination became more thorough than before.

Therapeutics had its advances too when William Withering (1741–1799), a physician of Birmingham and student from Edinburgh, published his *Account of the Fox-glove* in 1785. He had heard from a country woman that decoctions of fox-glove would cure dropsy. (This was a term used for a variety of fluid swellings of many kinds, but in this instance presumably meant widespread oedema, which would be visible in hands and feet). He was a renowned botanist, having published *Botanical Arrangement of all the Vegetables* in 1776—another example of the penchant of the age to gather facts and systematize them. He found that fox-glove did indeed cure some forms of dropsy, though not others now known to be renal or malignant. Thus was digitalis introduced, and in various more refined preparations it is still used in the management of cardiac failure. Of course it required later advances in chemistry and pharmacology before digitalis could be characterized.

Another therapeutic technique was similarly discovered almost by chance, and that was vaccination against smallpox. Edward Jenner (1749–1823) was a country practitioner in Gloucestershire, and a pupil of John Hunter's. He learned from country folk and a farmer called Benjamin Jesty that dairymaids rarely contracted smallpox, though they did become infected with cowpox from their herds. In one outbreak of smallpox, which then had a nearly 100 per cent mortality, Jesty did in fact inoculate some members of his family with cowpox to prevent the major disease affecting them. Jenner too carried out the appropriate inoculations on several patients and found they were not affected in serious epidemics. This he did at the instigation of John Hunter, who when Jenner told him of what he believed about inoculation with cowpox, replied 'Why think. Why not try the experiment?' This shows just how far medicine had progressed in its thinking. Experiment was to be added to observation, as Harvey had shown long before.

In 1798 Jenner published *An Inquiry into the Causes and Effects of Variolae Vaccinae* (*Figure 8.2*). It is of interest to note that Jenner was not the first to vaccinate, for Lady Mary Wortley Montagu, on a visit to Turkey, had had her

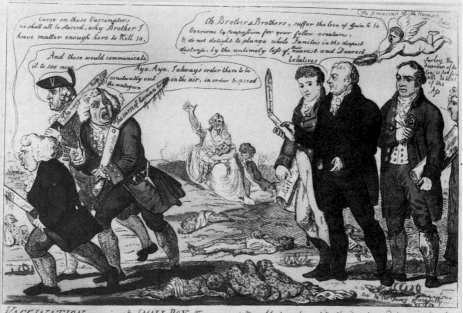

Figure 8.2 Coloured etching by I. Cruikshank, c1808. Caricature of vaccination. (Reproduced by courtesy of the Wellcome Institute Library, London)

3-year-old son inoculated in 1718, and later in 1721 her daughter had been inoculated in England. And there were other instances in other parts of the world, including Boston, in the USA. This shows how long it may take for a new idea and method to be adopted widely, even when in medicine it is efficacious. It is now remarkable that in the 1980s the disease of smallpox has been banished in all parts of the world. This immense achievement attained through international co-operation owes its origin to the education of the medical profession by Jenner nearly 300 years ago. Of course, as would be expected, the technique was vigorously resisted by many eminent doctors of the time, but positively demonstrated truth will usually triumph, given time. It could hardly have been foreseen that this method of vaccination would ultimately lead also to the modern successes of immunology, emerging in understanding of infection, inflammation, autoimmune diseases and the control of the mechanisms that cause rejection of tissue grafted from one individual into another. It is this knowledge that has made transplant surgery possible.

Surgery, anatomy and biology swept ahead in the hands of John Hunter (1728–1793), who was one of the great surgeons of all time. No doubt there have been many surgical practitioners his equal in operating, but few to vie with him in scientific enterprise in his subject. He came from Scotland to London in 1748 to join his brother William, the most eminent obstetrician of his day, a well-known surgeon, and founder of the famous Windmill Street anatomy theatre. It was with him that his brother John learned and taught, and he learned surgery under the tutelage of Cheselden and Pott (*see below*). He had a short spell in the army where he learned about gunshot wounds. He introduced the operation of tying arteries in healthy tissue above an aneurysm (a pulsating swelling of an artery caused by weakening of its walls by disease). This alone saved many lives and limbs. He added several observations in anatomy and tirelessly conducted animal experiments of all kinds. For this purpose he kept a menagerie at his home on the then outskirts of London, at Earl's Court. It is for this experimentation that he is chiefly revered now, for it was in the Harveian tradition and started surgery as a scientific discipline as distinct from being a rude craft, based in some degree on rule-of-thumb and experience. He amassed a wonderful series of anatomical and biological specimens, about 13 000 of which became the basis of the Hunterian Museum of the Royal College of Surgeons of England. Unfortunately much of this was destroyed by bombs during the war of 1939–45. Regrettably too, many of his notes and writings were destroyed by his brother-in-law, Sir Everard Home. This stupid man filched some of the work for various lectures and writings of his own and then burned the originals.

In the course of his experiments Hunter inoculated himself with pus derived from a patient suffering from venereal disease. In this way he contracted both gonorrhoea and syphilis. The two were not distinguishable then. Nor did this experiment help differentiate them, though Hunter described the natural history of the diseases as they affected him, and delayed the treatment (probably with mercury) so that he could make his observations. Towards the end of his life he suffered from angina pectoris, and feared that because of this he was at the mercy of anyone who irritated him. This is not surprising since he was a somewhat irascible and uncouth, even generally uneducated man, though warm hearted and generous to others. These characteristics, however, did not extend fully to his brother, William, with whom he fell out in an argument over priority in a discovery. This was an unfortunate, even silly, episode for each brother owed much to the other. But there

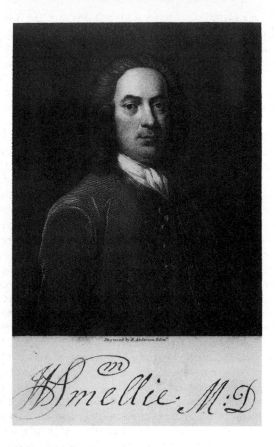

Figure 8.3 William Smellie [1697–1763].
(Reproduced by courtesy of the
Wellcome Institute Library, London)

is no guarantee that great men in one sphere of human life shall not be
pusillanimous in others.

The works of Hunter of most importance were *Natural History of the Human
Teeth* (1771), *On Venereal Disease* (1786), *Observations on Certain Parts of the
Animal Economy* (1786), *Treatise on the Blood, Inflammation and Gunshot
Wounds* (1794). As with many others, despite the clarity of his thinking in some
problems, he also carried in his mind some useless lumber from the past, especially
in the direction of vitalism—that is, that there is some special biological force as
distinct from those of chemistry and physics. The fact that the great have
weaknesses which all display in their humanity is endearing to those never likely to
reach the peaks of eminence.

A further important aspect of John Hunter is the number of his pupils whom he
inspired. They include Jenner, Abernethy (Hunter's successor), Astley Cooper,
Cline and Physick. This last was an American, who graduated at Edinburgh in 1792
and finally became professor of surgery in Pennsylvania. He carried the Edinburgh
and Hunterian principles with him and was a major founder of scientific surgery in
the USA.

William Cheselden (1688–1752) was a surgeon at St. Thomas's Hospital in
London. He devised an operation for stone in the bladder, through an incision
made in the perineum. It took him only about 90 seconds to perform! This was an

enormous boon in the days before anaesthesia. There was a premium on fast operating. In 1733 he published his *Osteographia*, a superb work on osteology, together with some illustrations of diseases of bone. It remained in use for many decades. He was yet another polymath for he designed a bridge which was built over the river Thames.

Percival Pott (1714–1788) was a surgeon at St. Bartholomew's Hospital in London. He sustained a fracture of the leg in a fall, but it was not the one of the ankle that now bears his name. He contributed works on hernia, head injuries, hydrocoele (swelling of the scrotum), fistula-in-ano (abnormal communication between the lower bowel and the skin of the perineum), fractures and dislocations, cancer of the skin of the scrotum in chimney-sweeps (another occupational disease) and tuberculosis of the spine causing paralysis by involvement of the spinal cord. The list is interesting, as is that of Hunter's works, for it shows the general state of the art of surgery. There was still no surgical invasion of head, neck, thoracic or abdominal cavities, despite much anatomical and pathological knowledge of these hidden areas. Surgery had, with a few exceptions, to remain confined more or less to the surface of the body until the advent of anaesthesia.

This work is too brief to be able to follow the history of the specialties in surgery and medicine, but it is worthy of note that Jacques Daviel (1696–1762) extracted the lens of the eye when it had become opaque through cataract, and he performed the operation on several hundred occasions with good results. William Heberden (1710–1801) described night-blindness (now known to be due to deficiency of vitamin A). It was he who described the bone nodules that occur on the fingers in some forms of arthritis. In ear, nose and throat surgery the mastoid was first opened surgically for abscess by Jean-Louis Petit in 1736. During the rest of the century this operation became more frequently performed.

The eighteenth century brought a revolution in obstetrics, mainly through dissemination of knowledge about the forceps. This demonstrates very forcefully the impact of new technology and invention on the general progress of a subject. The forceps demanded a new way of thinking, of observation, investigation and experiment in the problems of childbirth. There were many men who rose to this challenge of the new instrument, now no longer secret and belonging to the Chamberlen family. One of its numerous members retired to Woodham Mortimer Hall in Essex, to the north-east of London. There he died in 1683, and his widow gathered together his midwifery instruments and secreted them under the floor-boards of the attic. They remained there until discovered by chance in 1813. The discovery showed how the instrument had developed in various hands. The forceps became known to the medical public by a slow process of diffusion. Three doctors living fairly close to Woodham Mortimer learned of them by means unknown, but perhaps by meetings with Chamberlen and talks among themselves. Edmund Chapman, one of these three, published his *Essay on Midwifery* in 1733. In a second edition of 1735 he illustrated the forceps and described their use. Interestingly, he shows a pelvic curve on the blades. (The forceps originally had a cephalic curve to surround and hold on to the fetal head, and there were later some with straight blades. However, it has been deemed best if the blades also fit the curved birth canal of the mother, partly to make traction on the head more effective, and partly to minimize injury to the maternal soft tissues.) It was thought by some students of obstetric history that at first the blades were straight and that the pelvic curve was introduced later by Levret in France. But Chapman showed that the curve was in the original invention. He became so well known that he moved from Essex to practise in London. The other two doctors concerned in making the forceps known were William Giffard and Benjamin Pugh, both of whom wrote about them.

A point of interest is that in one case Chapman lost the pin, which locked the two halves of the forceps together at their cross-over point, in the sheets of a patient whom he was delivering. It will be remembered that the obstetrician of those days had to work entirely by touch, and was not allowed to see his patient's perineal region. He pressed on despite this mishap and to his surprise found that the instruments worked just as well without the pin. Over subsequent years the pin was left out of the design and now there is only a slot into which each blade reciprocally fits. In the hands of William Smellie this became known as the English lock.

William Smellie (1697–1763) is known as the Master of British midwifery (*Figure 8.3*). He came from Scotland, lured by rumours of the forceps. He went to Paris but found he could learn little there so returned to London in 1739. He set up a school of midwifery for doctors near Leicester Square. He and his pupils cared for poor women in the immediate vicinity, and all of them learned the use of the forceps. In his book *A Treatise of the Theory and Practice of Midwifery* of 1752 he laid down the rules for the safe use of forceps, which have been followed ever since. But the whole book is full of sound common sense and careful practice; and just as Hunter, another Scot, set surgery on its modern way, so did Smellie do the same for obstetrics.

It was because of Smellie that William Hunter (1718–1783) too came south from Scotland. He studied under Smellie and Dr James Douglas, whose name is still eponymously attached to the pouch of peritoneum in the female pelvis. From these two teachers William Hunter learned to be an obstetrician and an anatomist, which careers he followed with outstanding success. He prized his position as a teacher and especially as a 'breeder of anatomists'. He produced *The Anatomy of the Human Gravid Uterus* in 1774 (*Figure 8.4*), though Smellie had antedated him with his *Set of Anatomical Tables* of 1754. These were nothing like as complete as Hunter's which is still a most remarkable work.

These medical users of the forceps were vehemently attacked on many sides, and particularly by the local midwives. Some very unpleasant invective was bandied about, and these forerunners of obstetricians were dubbed man-midwives. They had tremendous obstacles to overcome in being accepted. There was still much prejudice about men appearing at all in the labour room. Yet they triumphed and it is perhaps not too much to claim that the obstetric forceps has been the most beneficent instrument ever designed. Used world-wide, they have preserved the lives of millions of mothers and babies and prevented untold suffering in childbirth. Of course, as with any other advance, it is possible to point to disadvantages and misuse and damage caused by them. But this pales into insignificance alongside the good they have brought about.

Following Smellie in his midwifery school was John Harvie, who described in 1759 a method of delivering the placenta that did not involve inserting a hand into the uterus through the vagina. This too must have saved untold lives, for the older method was fraught with the risks of infection and death from sepsis. And another enormous help in labour came from Fielding Ould (1710–1789) of Dublin, who popularized the operation of episiotomy in which an incision is made through the tissues of the perineum to make it easier for the baby's head to emerge.

Infection following childbirth, puerperal fever, killed many mothers. In 1773 Charles White (1728–1813) of Manchester, England, wrote on the fever and

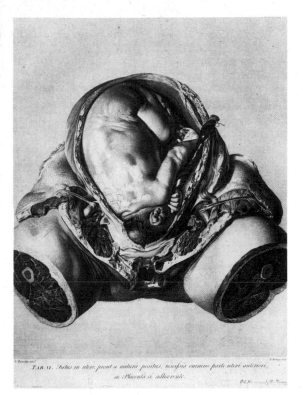

TAB VI. Foetus in utero, prout a natura positus, resectis omnino parte uteri anteriori, ac Placenta ex adhaerente.

Figure 8.4 From W. Hunter, *Anatomia uteri humani*, Birmingham 1774. (Reproduced by courtesy of the Wellcome Institute Library, London)

advocated cleanliness of patients, attendants and tools, as well as fresh air. This might almost be counted as the first steps towards asepsis, for general cleanliness in the eighteenth century left something to be desired. He characterized too the deep venous thrombosis that can follow childbirth and cause the massive swelling of the leg called 'white leg' or phlegmasia alba dolens. In 1790 he helped to found St. Mary's Hospital in Manchester. And another who was ahead of his time was Alexander Gordon of Aberdeen. In 1795 he showed that some midwives and some doctors seemed to carry puerperal fever to their patients, while others did not. But the mystery of the spread of infection had to wait for the advent of bacteriology in the next century.

In embryology was Casper Friedrich Wolff (1733–1794) of Berlin, whose *Theoria Generationis (Theory of Generation)* of 1759 supported Harvey in the ideas of epigenesis in which tissues and organs are deemed to differentiate and develop rather than be preformed only to grow in size in the fertilized egg. He came very close to recognizing the three germ layers from which the embryo is differentiated.

Partly as a result of the improved midwifery of the times the population slowly began to rise in England and Wales. In 1701 the numbers were about 5½ million, with the population of London being about 670 000. And one appalling statistic is that about 75 per cent of all children born died before they reached the age of 5 years. This was mainly because of infection, often based on malnutrition due to poverty. By 1800 the mortality for children below the age of 5 had dropped to about 40 per cent, and the total population was about 9 million. During the eighteenth century there was a shift of population to the cities and towns. The Industrial

Revolution is conventionally dated from about 1760. It was based partly on the mechanization of manufacturing processes by Watts' steam engine (1765), Arkwright's water frame (1769), Hargreaves' spinning jenny and Crompton's mule (1779), all of them of importance in the burgeoning textile industry. Although crowding into inadequate accommodation in slums in insanitary conditions, with killing infections likely to be rife, would seem to be totally disadvantageous, it is by no means always so. Incomes and the availability of food may increase so that malnutrition and resistance to infection may be ameliorated. The fact is that about 1790 the birth rate in London for the first time passed the death rate. There were probably many complex reasons for this, but better social conditions gradually arose, and there was concern for the people on a scale not previously known.

Street lighting was introduced in London in 1734. During 1761–5 various private Acts of Parliament brought in rating for houses, and the money was used to improve the environment. Moreover, Wesley's Methodism, with its concern for welfare of the people, gathered strength in London as early as 1738 and was fully established as a religious and social force by 1760. Rousseau's *Social Contract* was published in 1762. The Royal Humane Society was working in 1777 and Eden wrote on *The State of the Poor* in 1797. The following year Thomas Malthus wrote his Essay on the *Principle of Population* and showed concern that population growth might outrun food supply, which is a spectre still haunting the world today.

This very brief survey is intended only to show that there were powerful social and political movements afoot which indirectly were improving the health and the physical and mental lot of the people. Medicine is in some ways only a peripheral factor in helping to bring this about. Yet medical and social concern was shown in the founding of many hospitals. They demonstrate interest in people and especially the poor. Among hospitals founded, in London, were the Westminster (1719), Guy's (1721), St. George's (1733), the maternity hospital which became Queen Charlotte's (1739), the London (1740), the Foundling Hospital (for abandoned and sick children) (1741), the Middlesex Hospital (1745) and lying-in beds in that hospital (1747) (the first in the world in a general hospital), City of London Maternity Hospital (1750), the General Lying-in Hospital (1765), and there were dozens of others in the British Isles and round the world in Europe and America. The maternity hospitals are noteworthy as yet another by-product of the invention of the obstetric forceps. Moreover, there was a new spirit abroad about the place of women in society and their contribution to it. It was shown by the founding of these hospitals, in women's meetings and in literature, for this was the age of novels about women. Among them were Defoe's *Moll Flanders* (1722) and *Roxana* (1724), Richardson's *Pamela* (1740) and *Clarissa* (1747), Fielding's *Amelia* (1751) and many others. And at the end of the century in 1792 Mary Wollstonecraft produced her *Vindication of the Rights of Woman* whose title alone demonstrates how far the women's movement had progressed. This is borne out too by the fact that two now famous women novelists—Jane Austen and Fanny Burney—were writing towards the close of the century.

The growing enlightenment of attitudes towards other people extended to the mentally ill. The Retreat at York was founded in 1793 with the aim of caring for patients with humanity. That this was not an isolated phenomenon was shown when Philippe Pinel (1745–1826) struck off the chains of insane people at Bicêtre in 1798.

There was a background of war during much of the eighteenth century and this too had repercussions on society, its health and medicine in general. The battles were waged round Europe, with various alliances of the British with Holland and

Spain against the French, and then they were transferred to Canada and the United States, and on to the defeat there of the British in the War of Independence. And there were battles in the West Indies too where thousands of British soldiers died, often from epidemic infections. Then in 1789 came the French Revolution with its physical and intellectual consequences for much of Europe and especially Britain.

With the army was Sir John Pringle (1707–1782), yet another Scotsman from Edinburgh and Leyden. It was at the battle of Dettingen in 1743 that he suggested to the French commanding officer that the hospitals on each side should be respected and not attacked. This agreement and convention has been accepted ever since between warring armies. It is out of thinking like this that the Red Cross organization has arisen, to carry out its errands of mercy world-wide. In 1752 Pringle published *Observations on the Diseases of the Army* which introduced concepts of barrack-room ventilation and good sanitation with latrines. Even earlier, in 1750, he had written on gaol fever, usually now thought to be typhus, and made similar recommendations conducive to public health.

For the navy too there was a great doctor, James Lind (1716–1794), who in 1753 wrote *A Treatise on the Scurvy* (*Figure 8.5*). This disorder is now known to be due to deficiency of vitamin C. It was very prevalent among sailors on long voyages at sea when fresh foods, especially vegetables and fruit, ran out. Since the first signs of the

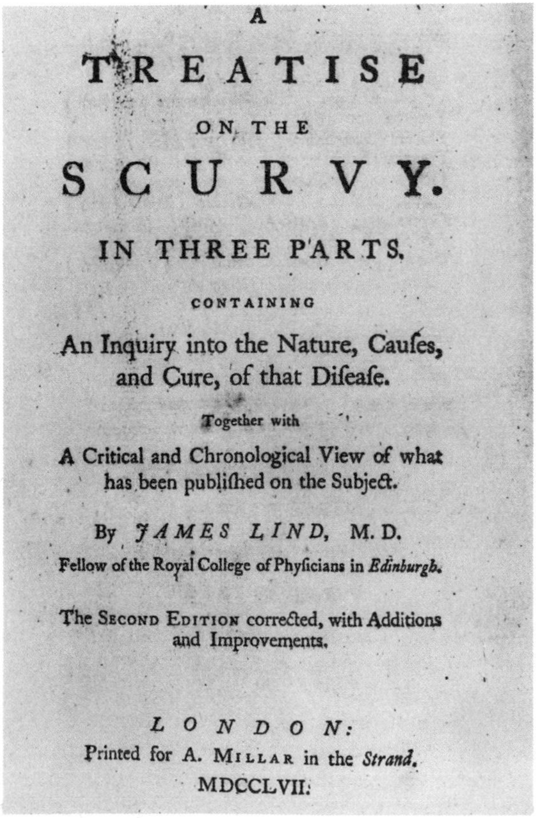

A

T R E A T I S E

ON THE

S C U R V Y.

IN THREE PARTS,

CONTAINING

An Inquiry into the Nature, Causes, and Cure, of that Disease.

Together with

A Critical and Chronological View of what has been published on the Subject.

By *JAMES LIND*, M.D.

Fellow of the Royal College of Physicians in *Edinburgh.*

The Second Edition corrected, with Additions and Improvements.

L O N D O N:

Printed for A. Millar in the *Strand.*

MDCCLVII.

Figure 8.5 James Lind. *A Treatise on the Scurvy.* (Reproduced by courtesy of the Wellcome Institute Library, London)

disease may be bad temper, scurvy has been implicated as a possible cause of mutinies, though obviously there were more likely causes too. Lind recommended the use of citrus fruits to be given to sailors and in fact it was limes that were issued, and ever after British naval sailors have been known as 'limeys'. Limes are not particularly anti-scorbutic, but they serve and as a result scurvy among sailors began to diminish. This was really the first observation to be made of a deficiency disease. It had good practical effect on Captain Cook's voyages of exploration, during the course of which he found Australia in 1770. There was very little illness and only one death among his seamen when many might have been expected. Lack of vitamin C tends to predispose to infections of many kinds, which in the close confines of a ship may be serious and even fatal.

After leaving the navy Lind practised in Edinburgh from 1748. In 1758 he became physician to the naval hospital recently built at Haslar near Portsmouth, a major naval base. The building had been begun in 1754 and another such hospital was started at Plymouth in 1758. These were responses to the almost constant wars at sea of the century, and the need for keeping sea lanes open, with their consequent results in injury and illness in sailors. The Seven Years War against France began in 1755, demanding much traffic across the English Channel and the western North Sea to the Low Countries.

The significance of these advances in military and naval medicine is that they show a special interest in the environment of people and how they are accommodated, cared for and fed. The fact is that this was and is done to maintain efficiency in the armed forces, but from this come ideas that are the very basic of public health and hygiene, and of occupational health in civilians. There is constant and continuing interplay of concepts and practices between all apparently separate branches of medicine, and between medicine, society and science. It is historically perhaps more easy to recognize in the eighteenth century which seems especially to demonstrate the beginnings of modern medicine and science.

Newton picked up many threads from the past, added to them and wove them in a different way. He is the paradigm of a new way of thinking. The people of the eighteenth century exploited this novelty in a variety of ways, some of which have been the subject of this chapter. The pace was quickening, especially in application of what had been theory.

By the end of the eighteenth century physics and chemistry were establishing themselves. Their technologies were beginning to have some slight use in medicine and biology. The microscope was used in these subjects, and so was the thermometer, but only sporadically. Digestion was being studied as in a chemical laboratory by taking salivary, gastric and pancreatic secretions and mixing them with food in glass vessels. Analogies were being drawn between physican and chemical phenomena and those of physiology. Some bodily processes were definitely shown to be of physicochemical nature. Measurement was becoming an order of the day in length and mass. It imbued the work of Stephen Hales and therefore came into physiology. Anatomy and pathological anatomy, sciences basic to medicine, began to be recognized as such, whereas it had been possible previously to practise empirically without using them much.

There came a more pervading interest in understanding as well as in doing. This is a real beginning of professionalism. The practice of a profession always implies knowledge of its theoretical basis, and then this was increasingly visible. Clinical investigation advanced because there was better observation, recording and classification of diseases. They became more readily recognizable in diagnosis to a greater number of doctors. Some illnesses could be crudely interpreted in the light of pathology. And there was the invention of percussion to increase the basis on which clinical information could be obtained. Therapy still had to be empirical, but brought vaccination and digitalis, both of which had to wait for later explanation of how they worked. But this too is commonplace enough in the progress of technology and science. Recurrent phenomena have to be observed at first before there can come the reasons why they recur.

Surgery and obstetrics began their modern progress in this century. The first imported experiment and put surgery on its way. The second was based on a new and revolutionary technology—the forceps. There is no single royal road to be followed in the progress of a practical art (science) such as medicine. And health depends on more than clinical practice can offer. This is shown by the advances made socially, which had their offshoots in hospital provision and the improvement in the environment, especially shown in the army and navy, and in attitudes to women, the poor and the mentally ill.

The founding of institutions may properly be seen as public responses to needs felt at the time. This is so with the building of hospitals and the start of many medical schools, especially those of Edinburgh and Glasgow, which made such great contributions, through their students, and whose influence spread far and wide in Europe and America. Their traditions remain alive even though now transmuted and transferred to numberless similar schools everywhere. In the relative simplicities of the eighteenth century it is easier to see the achievements of various institutions because they were new and fewer than they are now. The later vast increase, by its very size, seems to have led to dilution, but is better seen as diffusion to a vast variety of enterprises for the good of many more people. And in this matter of education, whether formal or informal, the means of communication must not be forgotten. Latin was displaced as the only vehicle of communication between the *cognoscenti* in the eighteenth century. The loss of a common language by the use of many vernaculars was offset by the great numbers who could benefit from education, and so use knowledge for more and more people. The numbers of books and journals increased greatly at this time. Moreover there were movements too in primary education so that more and more people could be in contact with the various worlds of ideas and learning through reading. There is an interweaving of myriad strands from many areas of endeavour and thought leading to better health and welfare of the people at large. In the contemplation of the history of medicine, this general background must not be forgotten. It is often of more importance to the theme than medicine itself, and it explains some of the progress in medicine, which responds to as well as stimulates the societies in which it operates.

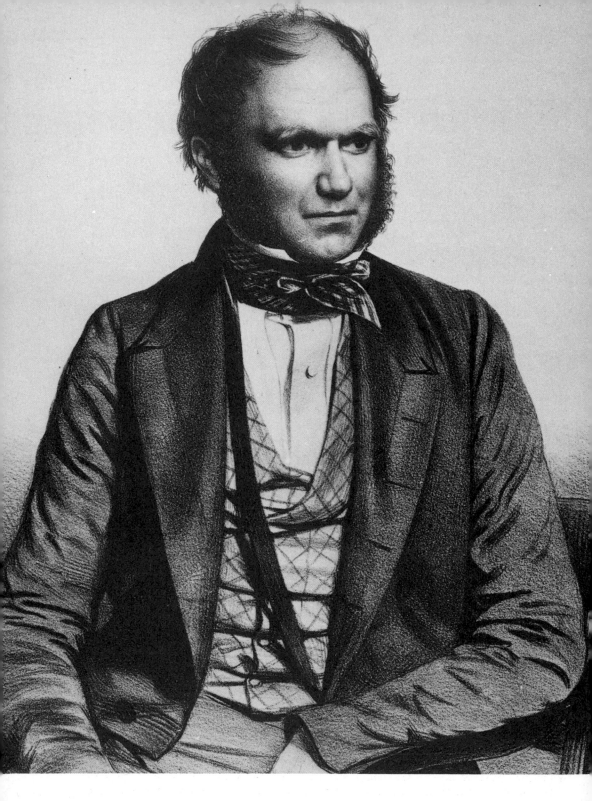

Charles Robert Darwin [1809–1882] (Reproduced by courtesy of the Wellcome Institute Library, London)

Chapter 9

Darwin's century (Nineteenth)

The nineteenth century is almost impossible to characterize in a slogan word or a few short sentences, So much was going on in industry, science, technology and medicine. All were founding the world as we know it now. Whereas in earlier centuries it seems possible to discern the large movements taking place in thought and action, this becomes more difficult as the present is approached. The welter of detail seems to become more important for fear of missing out something of present significance. It is easier to see the wood in remoter times, while the trees are more obtrusive in later ones. The historian, especially the amateur, has to be eclectic (so does the scientist) because of the large amounts of material available.

At the beginning of the century the aftermath of the French Revolution still dominated the scene politically, and it shaded off into the Napoleonic Wars waged all over Europe and on to the southern shores of the Mediterranean. The battle of Waterloo was in 1815. There was a British Army fighting in India and Afghanistan in the 1840s. The Crimean War began in 1854 and ended 2 years later. The American Civil War ran from 1861 to 1865. The Franco-Prussian War was fought in the 1870s, and at the end of the century in 1899 the Boer War in South Africa began, ending in 1902. There was a jostling for power in the western world and for the establishment of colonies. The driving force was the Industrial Revolution. Manufacturers needed outlets for their products, now being produced in quantity, and they needed raw materials, often from overseas. They produced wealth by which a nation could afford to put armies in the field and navies at sea. At that time wealth invested and also generated abroad needed armed protection, which it received. This was the capitalist system in full flood. It was scarcely questioned by the majority. It was the way things were ordained, probably by the higher wisdom of God. There need be no present sanctimony about this. Every age is blind to evils that later generations see. It is certain that the same is true now.

To work the mills, mines, and the industries based on machines, people were needed in ever-increasing numbers. In all countries populations rose. In this, medical advances had little if any part to play. Maternity hospitals were comparatively few and far between, and so had small impact on the rising birth rate and reduction of mortality at birth. Infectious diseases rampaged and nothing effective could be done about them medically. People were herded in slums with inadequate sanitation and impure water supplies, and conditions at work were similarly insanitary, with men, women and children working long hours in appalling

91

conditions. Poverty was often extreme and contrasted with the great wealth of a few manufacturers, mine owners and landed gentry. The death rate was high and expectation of life short. Yet death rates were smaller than birth rates, and survival rates for the younger age groups were higher than before. It is a surprising paradox. In 1801 the population of England and Wales was 9 million and rose to 10½ million by 1811. By 1911 the UK population (England, Wales, Scotland and Northern Ireland) was 42 million. Between 1815 and 1871 the population of Great Britain (England, Wales and Scotland) doubled from 13 million to 26 million. The drift from country to towns and cities, seen everywhere, is shown by the fact that the population of London was 1.25 million in 1820 and 3.25 million by 1871. These changes, repeated all over the western world, show that this century was a time of vast social upheaval, bringing in its train alteration in every aspect of health, medicine, science and the full range of society's endeavours and enterprises. Medicine and the sciences cannot be understood in isolation from this panoramic background.

The functions of such a complex, expanding society demand communication. The flow of information is a necessity for an industrial civilization and for science. Rapid travel, allowing more meetings of more people, with dissemination of knowledge, was adumbrated in 1815 when George Stephenson patented the first steam engine. This came into land transport with the opening of the Stockton and Darlington Railway in 1823, and the railway age had begun. The days of the stage-coach went forever. The age of sail at sea was similarly superseded when the first steamers plied between Dover and Calais in 1821. The total supersession of course took many more decades, but new methods always take a long time to diffuse into general use. The pace of that diffusion is dependent on the communication of knowledge to an ever-widening circle. The Penny Post began in 1840, and an Electric Telegraph Office was opened in London in 1846. The first radio communication between land and ships was made in 1898. Newspapers and journals became more popular and many were founded. Photography started in the 1820s and later improved immensely, so that communication became both verbal and visual. Societies were formed to disseminate and communicate information both to their members and to the general public. The British Association for the Advancement of Science began in 1831 for this purpose. With similar intent for medicine the British Medical Association started in the following year.

The list of new forms of communication could be made endless, but to no purpose here. This is enough to be reminded that the rate of advance in medicine and science is dependent on such technology and social organization. Knowledge is power. The larger the audience for knowledge, the more likely that it will be diffused for public benefit and that it will reach the ears of a few who will use, transmute and add to that knowledge. The nexus of society is totally dependent on information and communication as its essential substrate. The nineteenth century saw its start in the modern idiom. By contrast the earlier centuries show that immense effort was expended by only a few determined individuals to travel and communicate. Each journey was fraught with difficulties and even dangers. The travels and publications of the earlier heroes of this book, in search of knowledge and its advancement and communication, can now be seen to be incredible and almost superhuman.

Also in the background of the history of medicine must be counted some social movements, in the spirit of the century. There were many attempts to improve the lot of Man. Some evils were perceived in the social scene and serious efforts were made to ameliorate them. The press of the rising population and their various interest groups led to Reform Bills, slowly increasing the extent of the franchise. Political power was shifting from aristocracy, landowners and agriculture to the manufacturers, industrialists and even the working classes. Trade Unions for instance had their Acts to make them legal, after the establishment had too harshly punished the famous Tolpuddle Martyrs in 1834. In 1842 there was Shaftesbury's Mines Act which prohibited the employment of women and children underground. A later Act of 1847 limited the hours of work of women and children to not more than 10 hours daily. The Trades Union Congress was set up in 1869.

In 1876 there was an Elementary Education Act, making some early education compulsory for all, and there were many later amending Acts. There were also Public Health Acts, Housing Acts and Local Government Acts. Again this is all too brief, but it shows that despite many of the manifest drawbacks and inhumanities of the Industrial Revolution there was rising concern for humankind, at least in some quarters. That concern, and action arising out of it, was becoming recognized as a public necessity and duty. It is now known that many environmental factors, such as housing and education, have definite effects in the promotion of health and the prevention of disease. However imperfectly discerned, the recognition was growing that society as a whole must care for its weaker members, and that public organizations must be founded and controlled to make sure that various duties were carried out. The much maligned bureaucracy had begun in earnest, but if society is to function at all in its complexity then bureaucrats are essential, even though it is possible often to point to their inadequacies. But there is no known substitute for bureaucratic organization.

Unsurprisingly, this is the century in which Friedrich Engels (1820–1895), affected by his work in the textile industry of Manchester and Karl Marx (1818–1883) started communism, nor that they found the freedom to do so mainly in England. They expressed an important movement against prevailing adverse conditions for people in society. It is perhaps now seen as an extreme protest, but such extremes may express a more general movement of thought going on at a much less intense level.

The practitioners of science and medicine were inevitably prey to the general presuppositions of the age, as well as to those of the subjects they studied. In short they inherited a general and special culture, which they used and caused to evolve. The very word 'scientist' was coined for the first time in 1840 in Whewell's *Philosophy of the Inductive Sciences*. This new word marks a parting of the ways since it is a signpost in the growth of specialization. In previous times one person could encompass a great deal of general and special knowledge and be competent both in arts and in sciences. The knowledge explosion was still largely manageable by single well-stocked minds. The nineteenth century quietly killed the notion that the educated person could be on terms with all branches of knowledge.

In previous centuries many of the polymaths were doctors of medicine. They came to the subject through the classics and art, and studied the sciences of the day at their universities, adding clinical studies later. Indeed the universities were so organized that those who wished to study science often found it necessary to enrol with the faculties of medicine, under whose aegis the majority of sciences were, with perhaps the exceptions of astronomy and mathematics. Like the horse and sail the complete generalist departed for good in the nineteenth century, never to return as a practical proposition in human affairs. That fact still needs assimilation into education where there may be much tension between the generalists and specialists, the first group wishing for a calling back of what they see as the golden age. They cannot have read and understood history where examples of such harking back are commonplace and they fail in the face of reality.

In physics and chemistry the century saw continued progress, which was often spectacular and destined to be incorporated into medicine and its practice in the future. By 1804 John Dalton (1766–1844) had established the Atomic Theory, and his work was published a few years later. This propounded that all matter is made up of small particles which are indestructible. He showed that gases expand when their temperature is raised and that the total pressure exerted by a mixture of gases is the sum of the pressures that each would exert if present alone. It will be recalled that many before him, even those of classical Greek times, had suggested that the world was made of atoms, variously conceived in different philosophical systems. But Dalton drew the previous thoughts together and gave them an experimental scientific basis. And Avogadro (1776–1856) promulgated his hypothesis about 1811, which states that under equal conditions of temperature and pressure equal volumes of different gases contain the same number of molecules. Physics and chemistry were coming together, though both the Atomic Theory and Avogadro's hypothesis were much resisted at the time and became fully accepted only decades later. Now it is impossible to explain many biological and medical phenomena without recourse to physical chemistry and its concepts. Moreover, it is an essential basis of many therapies and the development of scientific pharmacology.

At another level the discoveries of the chemical elements went on apace. Humphry Davy found sodium and potassium in 1810, and did so by electrolysis, another interesting combination of physics and chemistry. In 1813 he produced the first work on agricultural chemistry. In 1828 Friedrich Wöhler (1800–1882) synthesized urea. This was epoch making, since urea was before this time known only as a biological or organic substance, and here it was produced in the laboratory by heating ammonium cyanate. In this way an organic substance was produced from an inorganic one without living material being responsible. The biological world was then made inseparable from the physical and chemical one. In retrospect this was an immense step, though it was only one among many others. The whole inorganic and organic chemical worlds were being opened up by thousands of researches, which included those into proteins, amino acids, plant materials and drugs. The industry shown and the results were tremendous. The hundreds of workers were rapidly changing the approaches to the nature of the physical and living worlds. Another step forward was provided by August Kekulé, who conceived of carbon chains but also of carbon rings, as in benzene and its many derivatives in organic compounds. Thus arose organic chemistry and its development into biochemistry.

Startling too were the researches into waves of many kinds. Clerk Maxwell (1831–1879) of Cambridge, and by some ranked only second in importance to Newton of the same university, deduced the presence of electromagnetic waves in 1864, and in 1873 published his *Treatise on Electricity and Magnetism*. This brought together the concepts of both, showing them often to be similar in nature, the one being convertible into the other under certain conditions. It demonstrated too that light is a form of electromagnetic wave, and not corpuscular, as Newton had thought (though the nature of light, as between these two ideas, is still not resolved). This has effects on the theory of vision and especially colour vision, and in therapy there have been many practical outcomes of electromagnetism. In 1895 Wilhelm Conrad Röntgen (1845–1922) (*Figure 9.1*) discovered what have come to

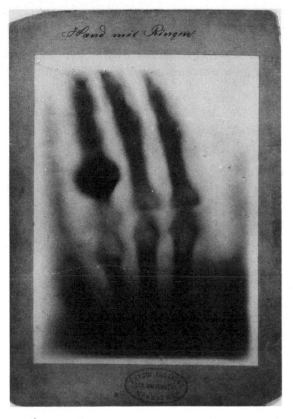

Figure 9.1 The hand of Frau Röntgen, photographed in X-ray by W. K. Röntgen, 22 December 1895. (Reproduced by courtesy of the Wellcome Institute Library, London)

be known as X-rays. Within a very few years these were being used in medicine for diagnosis, since it was realized that the rays would penetrate almost any material and cast a photographic shadow. At first this was displayed on a phosphorescent tube. A few months after Röntgen's discovery Henri Becquerel (1852–1909), in 1896, discovered uranium and its radioactivity, and in 1898 the Curies isolated radium from massive amounts of pitchblende which they had patiently worked on to reduce it to a few grams of the active substance. The wave revolution was truly begun. There were particles too (alpha and beta) which penetrated tissues. Not only were diagnostic radiology and radiotherapy started on their way, but the nature of physical matter was being understood quite differently from formerly. Particles dissolved into waves and waves disrupted atoms, which had been held to be indivisible. The atom began to yield up the secrets of its structure. Johnstone Stoney (1826–1911) first named electrons in 1894, applying the term to the beam of a cathode ray tube. The atom, instead of being static and indestructible, was now seen as a seething structure with a central core, positively charged, having outer shells of circling electrons which were negatively charged.

The idea of a static unchanging world disappeared for ever. Its very base, seemingly solid to common sense, was in flux all the time. This new concept was a very long way from that of Aristotle and Plato with its ideas of perfection and changelessness. By the nineteenth century nothing in nature was as it seemed. Everything was in dynamic motion. And still that idea informs and is part of all the sciences. To some extent it was put there by the Darwinian Theory of Evolution. In this sense biology was for the first time imported into a wider world of ideas. Yet it is more likely that the whole intellectual world of science was moving along similar parallel paths. The general idea of dynamism, change and evolution was in the minds of many, whose work in several fields were special exemplifications of the general perception. But it was, and is, an astonishing reversal of previous thought, allied with a burgeoning and sophisticated technology.

This wave revolution has emerged into radiology, radiotherapy, ultrasonography, isotopes, radioimmunoassay, nuclear magnetic resonance, non-invasive imaging techniques, phototherapy, spectroscopy, radio monitors for bodily functions as well as atomic energy and a variety of nasty destructive weapons. Nothing seems to be either wholly good or wholly bad.

Anatomy quietly forged ahead with deeper understanding and the naming of bodily parts. The microscope was increasingly used. Jacob Henle (1809–1885) of Zürick, Heidelberg and Göttingen, was a master of its use. Between 1866 and 1871 he produced his *Handbook of Systematic Anatomy* which covered all aspects of macroscopic as well as microscopic anatomy, and this was an innovation. Some regard him as the founder of histology. But it is difficult to separate anatomy from other subjects for which it formed the base. It was slowly changing from a pure science into an applied one. Its practitioners were not just specialists in the subject, but were physiologists, chemists, pathologists and clinicians. The specialization we know now had not been fully established though it was beginning. Great men occupied Chairs which often included two or more of each of these disciplines. Yet these researches in basic anatomy, esoteric though they may have appeared to be at the time, must not be derogated. The corpus of knowledge being gained had to await exploitation in practice when the techniques of anaesthesia, surgery and medicine had advanced sufficiently for nearly every detail of anatomy to be used. There is a general lesson to be learned here by those inclined to oppose expenditure on fundamental research. They may, in their shortsightedness, be unable to foresee immediate application of what is discovered, but later ages will. One of the values of the study of history is that it causes adjustments in concepts of time-scales and it induces patience. Not everything newly discovered comes to fruition in use in a single lifetime.

An unfortunate anatomist was Robert Knox (1791–1862) of Edinburgh. He was an inspiring teacher but he took little notice of where the bodies for dissection in his school came from. In 1829, William Hare, a lodging-house keeper, had one of his tenants die in debt to him. With Thomas Burke, another Irishman, he conceived of clearing the debt by sale of the body to Knox. This was done, but the result was that Burke and Hare were encouraged to proceed further in making money in this way, so they systematically murdered some of the denizens of the house and sold the bodies to the unsuspecting Knox, who was the subject of a great scandal which ultimately broke him, even though he was formally exonerated of any complicity in the murders.

Physiology exemplifies the way in which it is impossible to categorize medical practitioners in the nineteenth century. Charles Bell (1774–1842) was a superb surgeon and anatomist. He was a Scot who went to London and took over the anatomy school in Windmill Street. Later he was appointed to the Middlesex Hospital and then returned to Edinburgh as professor of surgery, by which time he had been knighted. But he is especially remembered because of *The Nervous System of the Human Body* (1830), in which he had determined the functions of the two roots of every nerve of the spinal cord—namely that the dorsal roots carried information about sensations and the ventral roots controlled movements. This is both anatomical and physiological knowledge, but the separation of the two always has been and remains artificial, for structure illuminates function and vice versa. Yet the separation into the specialties that we know now began with John Barclay (1758–1826) of Edinburgh, who professed only anatomy, and did not combine it with other disciplines.

At Bonn with Henle was Johannes Müller (1801–1858) who went to the Chair of anatomy and physiology in Berlin in 1833. Between 1833 and 1840 he produced his *Handbuch der Physiologie des Menschen* (*Handbook of Human Physiology*) which was a masterpiece of its time and made many new discoveries in the nervous system, in embryology and pathology and in the mechanisms of speech.

A professor of physiology at Königsberg University was Hermann von Helmholtz (1821–1894), who invented the first ophthalmoscope, which allowed inspection of the interior structures of the eye. This was a landmark since it extended the range of clinical observation into normal living anatomy and pathology. The outcome in the late twentieth century has been instruments that afford direct vision into all parts of the body—ear, nose, throat, upper and lower intestinal tract, the air tubes, vagina and uterus, the latter even when it is pregnant. And there are laparoscopes for looking directly into the abdominal cavity through a small incision, and thoracoscopes for similarly looking into the chest cavity. The inspection of the interior of the bladder and urethra in urological practice by appropriate visual methods is routine. Joints are inspected by arthroscopes.

All have come about as a result of improvements in the technology of light, illumination and optics, and Helmholtz first wrote on this in *Physiological Optics* of 1856–67. His work combined with that of Thomas Young (1773–1829) of London whose book *On the Mechanics of the Eye* was published in 1801. These two between them formulated a theory of colour vision.

It is noteworthy that the technology of the ophthalmoscope started off a new specialty of ophthalmology, in exactly the same way that the forceps initiated the study of obstetrics. This is another example of the interaction of technology with knowledge and specialization. By 1871 Helmholtz was professor of physics in Berlin where one of his assistants was Heinrich Hertz (1857–1894), whose name is now known to every amateur of radio and high-fidelity sound.

The outstanding physiologist of the century was undoubtedly Claude Bernard (1813–1878) of Paris (*Figure 9.2*). He made many discoveries in digestion, metabolism of glycogen and the vasomotor mechanisms. In 1865 he published *Introduction to the Study of Experimental Medicine*. This brought in the seminal concept of the relative fixity of the internal environment of the body. Darwin's work appeared in 1859 and this had emphasized the role of the external environment in evolution. Bernard's genius was to identify the fact that each cell of the body has an environment affecting its function, and that the sum of all these environments constitutes the internal environment. The major part of this is contributed by the chemical composition of the blood and tissue fluids bathing all the cells. Despite massive additions to and subtractions from the blood (by the gut and the cells of all organs) and secretions and excretions such as those of urine and the various ducted glands, the composition of the blood and tissue fluids remains more or less constant, without substantial variations quantitatively of each identifiable chemical substance.

In other words the animal body is able to preserve a relative chemical constancy in the face of change which is being imposed on it all the time. This is indeed a

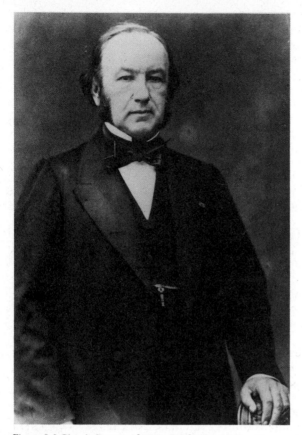

Figure 9.2 Claude Bernard [1813–1878]. (Reproduced by courtesy of the Wellcome Institute Library, London)

remarkable concept for it emphasizes the need for controls of the dynamism of the body. There have to be controls to damp down the otherwise potentially catastrophic effects of relatively massive change. The cells of the body can live only if their immediate environment is controlled within comparatively narrow limits. This therefore is all about control mechanisms. It raises questions about the causes of an increase in certain metabolic processes and bodily activities such as the heart and respiration rates, and what causes these same sorts of change to be decreased when they are excessive or are no longer needed for the bodily economy. The concept is still enormously fruitful in medicine and all its allied sciences, but further it has extended into much wider spheres in many human enterprises. The whole computer revolution of recent years as well as psychological and social concepts have been built on the ideas of positive and negative feedbacks, which are the essence of control mechanisms, first shown to be important by Claude Bernard.

Charles Darwin (1809–1882) is taken as the exemplar of this century because of his unifying synthesis of so many strands of thought and observation. His theories made sense of an immense range of scientific enquiry. They brought together many disparate discoveries, and so established links between them where none had been seen before. The unification and simplification threw a quite new light on many phenomena. Moreover his theories gave a new direction for future investigation, so that all the biological sciences were different conceptually after his time. Hypotheses were formulated in different ways and so were verifications and falsifications of natural processes. Today this still happens. Darwin's influence pervades every biological thought and experiment, even though this may be much modified by the passage of time and by new technology. It is amazing that one great theory, so general in its scope, can have had so many specific exemplifications in so many areas of human activity. A well-spring was tapped by Darwin which still flows, finds new paths and nourishes thought. His theory of evolution, in its generality, has not been falsified by evidence so far, despite attempts to do so. It will be recalled that Karl Popper, the scientific philosopher of the twentieth century, showed that the essence of the scientific method is that hypotheses are falsifiable. In resisting such falsification over a long period Darwin's achievement is nearly unique. There is of course no certainty that this will remain so.

Darwin tried medicine as a student and found that neither this nor other studies suited him. He was offered a post as naturalist on the voyage of the HMS *Beagle* to South America. It was during this that he observed the finches and turtles of the Galapagos Islands, and saw that although there was a basic pattern for each of these animals, the isolation of them on the islands had allowed, in some way then unknown, of quite marked variation from the norm. This, with much other later work, established Variation in species and he was also able to see that many variations in form and function were suppressed and held in check by Natural Selection. There were environmental pressures applied to every species, and much the most important of these was food supply and its scarcity. This idea he picked up from reading Malthus' *Essay on the Principle of Population* (1798). He took with him on the ship, which sailed in 1831, the recently published work by Charles Lyell on the *Principles of Geology*. This dwelt on the fact that the earth and its rocks and soils were not unchanging but were forever being acted on and affected by climatic changes—another example of the importation of the notion of change so typical of the nineteenth century. That the whole theory of evolution was abroad in the scientific community is also shown by the fact that Alfred Russel Wallace (1823–1913) on the opposite side of the world enunciated the same theory as Darwin. The two of them presented their papers to the Royal Society simultaneously, and Wallace most generously gave precedence to Darwin. This must be one of the most magnanimous gestures in the history of science.

The voyage of the Beagle ended in 1836, and by 1859 Darwin published his now celebrated *On the Origin of the Species*, but in full it is *On the Origin of the Species by means of Natural Selection or the Preservation of Favoured Races in the Struggle for Life*. The book caused a furore. Some senior clerics saw it as blasphemous. The redoubtable Thomas Henry Huxley vigorously defended its main thesis. Darwin himself virtually retired from the scene to his home at Downe in Kent where he continued his work, under the shadow of a mysterious debilitating illness, which had the merit of keeping him away from unwanted public controversy. In 1868 he extended his observations in *Variation in Animals and Plants under Domestication*. In 1871 there came *The Descent of Man* and *Selection in Relation to Sex*. By this time Man was not just a little lower than angels, he was at one with the subhuman animal world, even though he might choose to regard himself as its pinnacle.

It can now only be dimly realized what a revolution in thought this was. It opened up everything human to scientific investigation. Man was just as physical, chemical, biological as every other living thing, subject to the same sorts of process in endless cycles, recurrences, change and chains of being. Nothing about Man was thereafter sacrosanct and inviolate from the searches of science.

In 1858, the year before the *Origin*, Rudolf Virchow (1821–1902) produced his *Cellular-Pathologie* from Berlin. This established the basis of pathology in the cells of organs seen microscopically. Cells were the basis of normal and abnormal living. But we have seen how the whole medical and scientific world was edging towards this concept, and again it imported the ideas of process, dynamism and change in previously unperceived ways. And of course it is unfair to mention only Virchow for there were dozens of others pursuing similar courses of investigation and publishing their results in the newly founded journals. Many revered names added their mites to the sum of public knowledge, through their published articles. Because of rapid transit by rail and sea these journals reached an ever-widening readership.

Bacteriology began about this time with Louis Pasteur (1822–1895) (*Figure 9.3*), one of the most famous scientists of all time. His life was one of almost continuous discovery in every field he touched. For medicine the beginning was when he demonstrated that there was no spontaneous generation in fermenting or putrefying material, but that these processes were caused by bacteria which gained access from the air. And like Harvey his experiments were so simple and the results

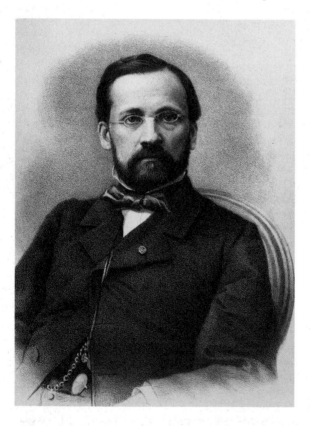

Figure 9.3 Louis Pasteur [1822–1895]. (Reproduced by courtesy of the Wellcome Institute Library, London)

undeniable. He showed that organisms were the cause of disease in silkworms, of fermentation in wine, beer and spirits, and of the fatal disease of animals—anthrax. The pasteurization of milk is named after him, and he is specially remembered for producing a vaccine against rabies, the fell disease caused by the bite of an infected dog (*Figure 9.4*). A Pasteur Institute was founded for him in Paris in 1889, and

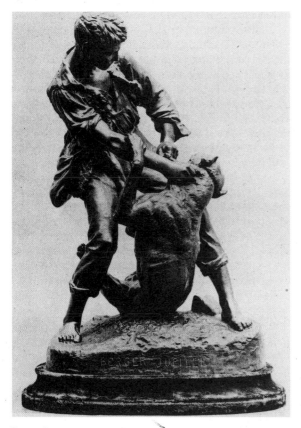

Figure 9.4 Statue at the Institut Pasteur of Jean-Baptiste Jupille fighting a rabid dog. Jupille was one of the first people to be inoculated against rabies. (Reproduced by courtesy of the Wellcome Institute Library, London)

similar institutes began all over the world and still remain. He triggered off a whole new science of immense importance and likely to remain so in medicine, science, technology and industry. He was a giant among giants of the time.

Having opened up the field, Pasteur was followed by many who applied and extended his work, in the tradition and pattern that has been emphasized before in this book. Robert Koch (1843–1910) was taught by Jacob Henle at Göttingen. He investigated anthrax and fully worked out its bacteriology. He perfected bacteriological methods of staining, fixing and culture, which, in essence, are still used. In 1882 he discovered the bacillus of tuberculosis, then one of the major killing and crippling diseases, and clinically often impossible to differentiate from others. He went on to make discoveries in many other bacterial diseases and brought in methods of sterilization. He is famous for the postulates he made for proving that a particular disease is caused by a specific bacterium: the organism must be found in all cases of the disease in question; it must be capable of isolation in pure culture in the laboratory; and when injected into an animal must reproduce the disease.

There were many others pursuing similar lines of investigation, among them being Friedrick Loeffler (1852–1915) (diphtheria) and Albert Neisser (1855–1916) (gonorrhoea) (both Germans), William Henry Welch (1850–1934) (gas gangrene) and Howard Taylor Ricketts (1871–1910) (typhus) in the USA. The list is very incomplete. And not only were these investigations concerned with the causes of disease, they began to lead to rational prevention and therapy. They revolutionized the practice of surgery under Joseph Lister.

Elie Metchnikoff (1845–1916) of Russia showed the importance of bodily defences by the white cells of the blood against attacks of infection. Often polymorphonuclear leucocytes can be seen under the microscope to have ingested bacteria into their cytoplasm where the organisms may be killed. This was the cellular defence. In addition it had been realized that some bacteria, especially those causing diphtheria, produce toxins to which the body produces antitoxins. So there is also a humoral or chemical defence. These notions helped on their way the concepts of bodily integrity which have led to the modern triumphs of immunology in the understanding of disease, and they have led also to the possibility of transplant surgery without rejection of foreign tissue. In 1891 Emil von Behring (1854–1917) in Berlin first treated a child suffering from diphtheria with the antitoxin and it was a great success. The medical treatment of infection then became a possibility in a specific sense, whereas before all that could be done was to prescribe rest, sleep, diet and non-specific measures or rarely to prevent them by vaccination (smallpox, Jenner; rabies, Pasteur). It is important to note how world-wide this new science was. Every country's scientists made their contributions, and the whole process was fuelled by the easier dissemination of information by publication and transport noted earlier.

From the present point of view medicine was making some progress in clinical investigation, as well as in understanding based on the natural history of disease and its interpretation in terms of bacteriology and pathology. Yet the outcomes in therapy were rudimentary, where the relative lack of success scarcely justified the arrogance of physicians, traces of which remain discernible. Jean-Nicholas Corvisart (1755–1821), physician to Napoleon, in 1808 popularized Auenbrugger's method of percussion, and he also wrote an *Essay on the Diseases and Organic Lesions of the Heart and Great Vessels* in 1806. He did this without the benefit of Réné-Théophile-Hyacinthe Laënnec's (1781–1826) discovery of auscultation. Laënnec's book of 1819 *Traité de L'auscultation Médiate* (*Treatise on Mediate Auscultation*) is an important landmark in clinical investigation. Sounds originating in the heart, lungs and other organs were known, for some may be heard at a distance from the body and some when the ear is directly applied to the skin, though the latter investigation was scarcely used. Moreover the sounds were not correlated with the lesions in the body cavities. Almost by chance Laënnec discovered that if he rolled up a paper tube and applied one end to the chest and the other to his ear, then bodily sounds were transmitted and could be interpreted.

The word 'mediate' was used to emphasize the interposition of the tube between observed and observer without the necessity (and indignity, as well as immodesty in examining women) of applying the ear directly. With a later edition of the book in

1826 the diseases of the chest and heart began to be categorized clinically and pathologically. For some time the stethoscope remained a monaural instrument (*Figure 9.5*) (as it still is in obstetrics for listening to the fetal heart) but soon became binaural in the sort of pattern known today, and without which no embryo doctor deems himself to be properly equipped. The word 'stethoscope' means inspection of the chest, and so is something of a misnomer. As with all new techniques the place of this one was hotly disputed at the time, but this reaction seems to be an historical necessity for everything really new in medicine. Like percussion before it, auscultation demanded fuller physical examination of the patient than was usual earlier. This was an immense gain in clinical method. Moreover it helped to pull together all the evidence arising from post-mortem examinations, pathology and bacteriology in the interpretation of disease in the patient.

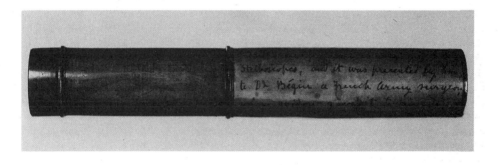

Figure 9.5 Laënnec's stethoscope. (Reproduced by courtesy of the Wellcome Institute Library, London)

In the 1820s an aural speculum was perfected and by 1896 Scipione Riva-Rocci, an Italian, building on much previous work, had produced an instrument for measuring the blood pressure, called a sphygmomanometer, much like the instrument in use daily now. An inflatable cuff is applied to the upper arm, while the doctor listens to sounds transmitted to the arteries below the constriction of diminishing pressure through a stethoscope. The fashion for measurement in clinical medicine was gaining strength. Prior to about this time medicine was qualitative and a matter of opinions. Hereafter it became increasingly quantitative.

In Ireland were great clinicians, among them being Robert James Graves (1796–1853) who described diseases of the thyroid gland, and his name is still given to exophthalmic goitre, which he wrote on in 1835. Contemporary was William Stokes (1804–78) and in the same hospital as Graves, who described with Robert Adams (1791–1875) a form of heart-block in 1826. There was also Dominic John Corrigan (1802–1880), who wrote on diseases of the aortic valve and the 'collapsing' pulse which incompetence of closure causes.

At Guy's Hospital, in London, were Richard Bright (1789–1858) and Thomas Addison (1793–1860) who in 1827 and 1855 respectively wrote on their work in renal and adrenal gland diseases. These were classics of clinical and pathological investigation. For some time too Thomas Hodgkin (1798–1866) was at Guy's and in 1832 described the disease with enlarged lymph glands still referred to by his name. Also in London was James Parkinson (1755–1824), who described his disease of the nervous system (paralysis agitans) in 1817.

In the USA William Beaumont (1785–1853), an army surgeon, had a patient, Alexis St. Martin, whose healed gunshot wound of the abdomen allowed of direct inspection of the interior of the stomach. Beaumont was able to observe many of the physiological changes of digestion and the vascular responses of the stomach lining caused by emotions. This might be counted as the start of psychosomatic medicine, bringing mind and body together in a continuum.

Surgery began a great leap forward because of the beginnings of anaesthesia and of bacteriology. Like advances in other disciplines the discoveries were world-wide, dependent on the work of many people, though now exemplified by a few eminent names. Anaesthetic gases, especially nitrous oxide and ether, had been known for some time when Horace Wells (1815–1848), a dentist of Hartford, Connecticut, USA, in 1844 induced a visiting lecturer on chemistry, Gardner Colton, to administer to him the 'laughing gas' (nitrous oxide) for the extraction of a tooth. The procedure was painless. (The name of laughing gas was given because it was used in fun as a party game in which people inhaled it and then felt strange while laughing a great deal.) Further experiments by Wells were not so successful and the administration of gas seemed unreliable.

Wells' partner in dentistry was William Thomas Morton (1819–1868), who moved to Boston, Massachusetts. He tried ether, which like nitrous oxide had been used for the party game of 'ether frolics'. In 1846 Morton administered ether to a patient of the surgeon, John Collins Warren (1778–1856), of the Massachusetts General Hospital. Again the operation was painless. (An Ether Dome at the MGH marks this historic event.) Unfortunately, Morton kept the nature of his anaesthetic secret—just as the Chamberlens had done with the obstetric forceps. He even coloured the liquid, but times had changed and he was the subject of odium.

A more pleasing sidelight is that it was Oliver Wendell Holmes (1809–1894) the famous literary figure of Boston, better known for his writings on the puerperal fever (for which see later), who named the new process 'anaesthesia'. The news soon reached London about the possibilities of anaesthesia, and at University College Hospital in 1846 Robert Liston (1794–1847) amputated through the thigh whilst the patient was under the influence of ether, and again the operation was painless. The young Joseph Lister witnessed the operation. It is impossible now to conceive how surgery could be practised without the boon of anaesthesia. It has allowed surgical intervention in all parts of the body with deliberate care, obviating the necessity for speed and haste, replacing it with scrupulous technique despite due expedition. The gain for patients is incalculable.

The story of anaesthesia was taken a little further by the famous obstetrician James Young Simpson (1811–1870) of Edinburgh (*Figure 9.6*). With colleagues he experimented convivially, after dinners given for them, on various substances to see whether they could be used as anaesthetics for the relief of pain in childbirth. He had already tried nitrous oxide and ether. Ultimately he lighted on chloroform, which when inhaled made some of his guests fall under the table. He was quick to try it out on women in labour and found it successful. There was a great outcry against the practice, led by puritanical clerics and their adherents, who (as with

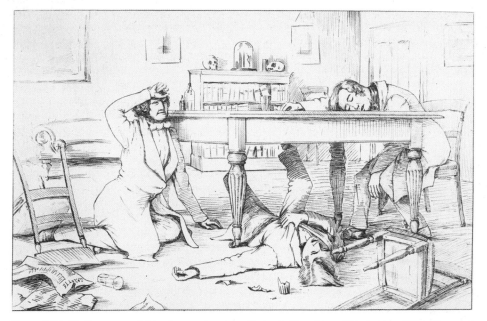

Figure 9.6 J. Y. Simpson and friends experiencing effects of chloroform, 4 November 1857. (Reproduced by courtesy of the Wellcome Institute Library, London)

many other advances) said it was not natural to interfere in this way, and they quoted the Bible as saying 'in sorrow shalt thou bring forth'. This criticism was finally silenced when the revered, moral and religious Queen Victoria accepted chloroform in two of her labours. It was administered by John Snow (1813–1858) who wrote *On Chloroform and Other Anaesthetics* in 1858. Thereafter pain relief in childbirth became respectable and has now advanced beyond all measure—though chloroform is no longer used, since there are some dangerous side-effects. Because of its use for the queen the method was known well into the twentieth century as 'chloroform à la reine'. Of course anaesthesia has changed its techniques and now a large number of products of modern pharmaceutical research are used, though the essentials as established in the mid-nineteenth century remain basically the same.

Surgery, in the early years of the century, made sporadic advances. Ephraim McDowell (1771–1830) of Danville, Kentucky, USA, performed the first ovariotomy, in 1809, in which a large ovarian cyst was removed from the abdomen. It was a complete success, though an extremely risky procedure at that time. His own reputation among the local townsfolk was at stake too, but the outcome silenced his critics. It has to be remembered that the operation was performed in his house without benefit of anaesthesia. He later operated on a further 12 patients, and eight recovered. Others, about the same time, did the operation independently or followed the lead of McDowell. This breaching of the peritoneal cavity of the abdomen was very remarkable, although it had been done very occasionally for a few centuries, especially with caesarean section. In general the mortality was so high that surgeons found discretion the better part of valour both for themselves and for their patients. This was why they tended to confine themselves more or less to the surface of the body.

Even the classic and courageous work of James Marion Sims (1813–1883) confirms this. He was the first to operate successfully on vesicovaginal fistula. This is an abnormal communication between the bladder and the vagina, caused by damage to the tissues during childbirth. Thereafter urine dribbles away continuously, making the sufferer's life a misery and causing all to shun her because of the smell always surrounding her. Sims worked in Alabama and saw black slave women with the disorder become outcasts and economically useless to their owners. In the grounds of his home he had a hut in which he housed some of these unfortunates and tried to help them by operating to close the hole in the vagina and bladder. He discovered the position in which to put the patient for operation, because if the woman is on her left side with the right knee drawn up towards her chest the vagina opens up, and this was very obvious where the pink skin of the vagina of his patients contrasted with the surrounding black. He used a bent spoon to draw the posterior wall of the vagina away from the fistula, which he repaired with the unabsorbable sutures of silver wire. In developing his technique he operated on his first patient 33 times before the leak was stopped. And again it must be remembered that this was all without anaesthesia. It shows how much suffering the injury caused for the woman to accept these many trials. In 1853 Sims moved to New York and 2 years later established the State Hospital for Women, the first such in the world, and so he started the separate discipline of gynaecology, perhaps the first surgical speciality, apart from ophthalmology.

Another surgeon, practising gynaecological surgery which was then the advancing subject, was Thomas Spencer Wells (1818–1897), who invented his forceps for the temporary control of vessels bleeding at operation. These have ridges on their jaws for grasping the tissues and a small ratchet on the handles which holds the jaws shut until the bleeding points can be tied with a ligature. He performed his first ovariotomy in 1858 and had many successes with the operation subsequently. He became President of the Royal College of Surgeons of England.

By the time of the advent of bacteriology and anaesthesia surgical technique of a kind was ready. It is essentially simple, needing scalpels, forceps, ligatures, needles and sutures, with various retractors to hold wounds open for access to various anatomical parts. Yet the simplicity of the tools does not disguise the boldness, courage, dexterity and skill of the surgeon, especially in pre-anaesthetic days. The pain then inflicted was a proper deterrent for all except the most desperate cases. There were also the twin terrors of haemorrhage and infection. If bleeding cannot be controlled, the patient inevitably dies, or, less than this, remains ill for a very long time. And whenever the skin is breached in trauma infection is almost invariably the rule. In fact surgeons referred to 'laudable pus' as evidence that all was going well.

It is impossible now to comprehend how surgeons could have been so deluded, but then they could have had no idea of how and why infection occurred. It must have seemed an inevitable and natural part of surgical intervention and of trauma. Then came Pasteur, and slowly the natural history of surgical and other infections was revealed. It was Joseph Lister (1827–1912), of Edinburgh and London, where he was professor of surgery at King's College Hospital, who first grasped the importance of Pasteur's work and realized its significance for wound sepsis. To try to kill the bacteria, which he suspected were in the air and all around the patient being operated on, he invented a spray of carbolic acid, so that there was a fine mist of this agent near the site of the surgeon's work. The results in the reduction of infection and sepsis were, for the times, near miraculous. Wounds healed cleanly, and in the jargon 'by first intention'.

It has to be remembered that operations were performed on almost any old table, there was draped furniture in the room, and surgeons, assistants, nurses and students wore their outdoor clothes. The surgeon might keep his jacket on and simply roll up his cuffs. The instruments were not sterilized. Even cleanliness was at a premium and surgical cleanliness was not conceived. Yet, as the word spread, antisepsis of the Listerian kind was practised in all the countries of Europe and the USA, and asepsis was gradually added to it, which finally all but replaced antisepsis. In the aseptic method everything possible is done to prevent bacteria getting into surgical wounds from the patient's skin, from the breath and hands of those in the operating theatre, by the sterilization of instruments, and by all changing into special clean clothes and wearing sterilized gowns and gloves. All of these changes took time to be introduced and to be practised widely all over the world, but now the methods are standard wherever surgery is practised.

Towards the end of the century anaesthesia allowed surgeons to develop operations for lesions in any part of the body. To these invasions the cavities of the head and thorax were somewhat resistant. They posed especially difficult problems of access to the diseased area and the supporting technology for operating on nerve, lung and cardiac tissue was not then available to offer solutions. This only came in the twentieth century. The abdominal cavity was much more accommodating for surgical intervention. Slowly the major abdominal operations were established in Britain, France, Germany, Russia and the USA. It is impossible in a short book even to list the names of those who contributed to this tremendous advance. Many of these are eponymously remembered in operations they invented, developed or popularized, just as anatomists in previous centuries had their names associated with structures.

There is much anxiety today about what has come to be called high-technology medicine, and this is allied with doubts about the ethics of performing certain operations, particularly those of transplantation, especially of the heart and liver. In addition there are critics of basic science research, which appears to have no practical immediate value. This just recounted story of surgery shows that anatomy was a science of little use for centuries until anaesthesia, bacteriology and surgery made it valuable. Moreover the abdominal operations, which are now standard and almost without risk, were originally high technology, had a high mortality, were experimental and had to have their efficacy confirmed or refuted by experience. This was especially so with appendicitis. The pathology of the condition was established by Reginald Heber Fitz (1843–1913) of Boston, USA. Charles McBurney (1845–1913), of New York, devised an incision to reach the affected organ, and others round the world 'experimented' with the problem. The results are now well known. The operation can be performed by the veriest tyro surgeon, speedily and easily, with small risk, and it has saved hundreds of thousands, possibly millions of young lives.

The same is true of operation after operation and will probably turn out to be true of the advanced ones now being criticized as of doubtful morality, outcome and applicability. History shows what the likely course will be. The pioneers will establish the methods and make them relatively simple; their teachings will diffuse to an ever-widening circle of surgeons, and the esoteric will become commonplace, so that doctors and patients will come to expect that these once rare operations will become available for more and more people. The present resistance will be overcome and the new techniques will be established, and perhaps, in their time, superseded also, like so many other ventures.

Obstetrics, too, quickly accepted the gifts offered by bacteriology and anaesthesia. In the forceps and caesarean section operations were the techniques for dealing with the problem of obstruction to birth. But they, and even normal labour inflicted pain, often of great severity. It is perhaps not surprising to find the obstetrician, James Young Simpson, in the forefront of the search for pain relief for childbearing women. Chloroform became widely used, and of course there was much use made of opiates for pain relief, but sometimes these had ill-effects on the babies. However, the really important change was in the thinking that made it right to seek for analgesics and anaesthetics for helping to overcome the pain of labour and obstetric operations.

Just after birth women are vulnerable to the horrors of severe haemorrhage, which until recent decades might be unstoppable and fatal. Heroic measures might be used, such as manually removing the placenta (or afterbirth) from inside the uterus, but this could make haemorrhage worse, or rupture the uterus, and even if the patient did not succumb she became very prone to infection, occasioned by the hand's invasion of the cavity and the anaemia due to the bleeding. Even without such catastrophes the woman shortly after giving birth is very prone to infection. Where the placenta has come away from the uterine wall is a raw, oozing area which is highly suitable for the growth of bacteria and consequent serious infection. This had been known for some time. In Vienna Ignaz Philipp Semmelweiss (1818–1865) knew that women begged not to be taken to the obstetric wards of the hospital, where they knew the death rate from puerperal fever was high. He showed that infection was particularly likely to occur in patients attended by students and doctors who had recently performed or attended post-mortem examinations on women dying of sepsis. He suggested that they carried the infection from the autopsy room to the women, and was reviled widely by the profession for saying so, even though he was right. It was in 1861 that he published *The Cause, Concept, and Prophylaxis of Puerperal Fever*. By then he had become professor of obstetrics in the University of Budapest, but he was unable to withstand the storm he had aroused and died insane, killed by the odium of a profession that would not look at the evidence and understand it. They had been told previously by Gordon of Aberdeen and by White of Manchester, but would not listen then.

In Boston, USA, Oliver Wendell Holmes was subjected to similar vilification. In 1843 he read a paper to the local medical society *On the Contagiousness of Puerperal Fever*. He advocated that obstetricians attending childbearing women should not also be associated with infected patients of any kind and should not be party to autopsies on infected bodies. Moreover he insisted that nails should be scrubbed with a brush and that the hands should be washed and rinsed in chloride of lime. The doctors were outraged and believed that this was an attack upon them and they responded with some vehemence and great acrimony. Holmes' reply that 'a gentleman with clean hands may carry the disease' did nothing to mollify the reaction. The statement shows how the profession totally (almost wilfully) misunderstood that the doctors' personal cleanliness was not under attack. They equated infection with dirt, which is still too common among those unaware of the implications of bacteriological knowledge.

The light shed by Pasteur and his followers, and by Lister with his, suddenly illuminated the terrors of puerperal fever and how they might be prevented by attention to the principles of antisepsis and asepsis. In Semmelweiss's time as many as 10 or more per cent of women having babies in some institutions died of infection. Often maternity hospitals and wards had to be closed because of the insistent mortality. In 1877 the General Lying-in Hospital, in south London, remained closed for nearly 2 years. Lister from the nearby King's College Hospital was called in to advise on what should be done, so he made his contributions to obstetrics directly, as he did to surgery. After his time the number of deaths from puerperal fever fell dramatically, but have virtually disappeared only with the coming of antibiotics in the mid-twentieth century.

There was some increased understanding of the sciences basic to obstetrics, and as always there was much interest in the early phases of development of the embryo. Caspar Friedrich Wolff's earlier *Theoria Generationis* (1759) was translated into German in 1812. Carl Ernst von Baer (1792–1876) in St. Petersburg, Russia, had established embryology by describing the germ layers more exactly than previously, but his famous contribution was to see the ovum (of a bitch) for the first time in 1827. This meant that fertilization could begin to be understood. And as with all subjects there were further discoveries, which came thick and fast. Yet in some ways dwarfing them all in significance were the researches of Gregor Johann Mendel (1822–1884) (*Figure 9.7*) into inheritance. He was a monk of Brünn (now Brno in Czechoslovakia) and his unlikely subjects for experiment were peas—some being green and wrinkled and some yellow and smooth. He carefully noted and recorded how these characters were passed on to progeny and was able to derive

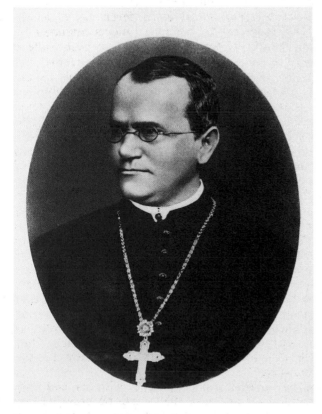

Figure 9.7 Gregor Mendel [1822–1884]. (Reproduced by courtesy of the Wellcome Institute Library, London)

general and mathematical laws about inheritance, applicable to the rest of the biological world. It matters little now that his sympathetic gardeners may have fudged some of the results, no doubt to please their master; his conclusions have been essentially borne out. Again the simplicity and incontrovertibility of the experiments has to be noted. The elegance rivals that of Harvey and Pasteur.

A surprising feature of the story of Mendel is that his work began in 1856, though not till 1865 did he communicate some of his results to the Brünn Society of Natural Science. They remained in the archives there until discovered in 1900, 35 years after publication, and after his death, by three botanists, pursuing similar paths to those of Mendel. Here at least was one scientist content to hide his light under a bushel, probably because neither he nor others fully appreciated what he had found and its significance for the future—yet another example of research in basic science having to wait for the right climate in order to come to practical fruition. Mendel in fact had read Darwin's works and made marginal notes in some of them, though there is evidence that the monk began his research before Darwin published. Indirectly, of course, Mendel was supplying the missing pieces in the jigsaw puzzle of Darwin's Theory of Evolution. The missing part was how Variation occurred in individuals of the species, on which Natural Selection could work to ensure survival of the fittest. The mechanism is genetic variation, produced by sexual reproduction, which we now know intermingles genes which force the animals or plants to reproduce certain characters in individuals—such as greenness, yellowness, smoothness and wrinkledness in peas! And moreover, these characters do not mix with each other to give (say) an intermediate yellowish green. They breed true—that is there is independent assortment of the genes and so little blending of characters. The basis of inheritance is dependent therefore on discrete units. And Mendel started it all in an amazingly seminal way. He prepared the path that has led to so much understanding, which has had practical outcomes in animal husbandry, in crop cultivation and in medicine.

Psychiatry in the modern sense began in the last decade of the nineteenth century with Sigmund Freud (1856–1939), of Vienna. The names of Adler and Jung in this new discipline should not be forgotten either. Freud had studied under Jean-Martin Charcot (1825–1893), the famous neurologist of Paris, who had a real interest in psychological phenomena in his patients. There were many others too in most parts of the western world who had similar concerns, but as in many other disciplines they were essentially recording and observing, and it was Freud's genius to give them a theoretical background which made some sense of what they saw. He brought understanding and also a method—psychoanalysis—which in a formal way had not been used before. The story of the full development of psychiatry belongs to the twentieth century, where Freud's influence has had its effects on literature and the arts, as well as on science and medicine. He brought some sort of order to that borderland between biology and sociology, though sociology as such did not then exist. Freud deserves to be ranked with Newton and Darwin for his theoretical insight which has turned out to be so fruitful in practice. It is not suggested, of course, that the theories of these three were or are acceptable in full in their original statements, but they each changed the direction of thought of their times in valuable ways. Here are examples of the remarkable interactions of speculation on a grand scale with practical sequels in science and technology, and indeed in many other human enterprises. If this relationship of great concepts with practicality is not grasped, then it is not possible to understand the nature of science. The lesser scientists than these giants too often restrict scientific thinking to the hillocks of thought, forgetting that the eminent pioneers have allowed them to glimpse the mountain peaks, which put their smaller worlds in context and give them order.

Following the flag in various colonial conquests in tropical and subtropical areas were several doctors with the armies. It was their job to try to keep the fighting forces healthy. Malaria was particularly rife and sometimes fatal. In 1880 Alphonse Laveran (1845–1922), serving with the French in Algeria, saw malaria parasites in the blood of an infected patient. The role of the mosquito in transmission was then suspected but not proved. Patrick Manson (1844–1922), a Scot, working in Hong Kong showed in 1877 that filaria worms were taken from the blood of patients with filariasis by a mosquito bite at night and that the organisms were handed on to others when the insect bit once more. In 1897 when he returned to London he founded the London School of Tropical Medicine. In that same year Ronald Ross (1857–1932) serving with the army in India showed the role of mosquitos in transmitting malaria. And a Cuban, Carlos Finlay (1833–1915) first suggested that yellow fever was similarly transmitted, though it was not till later that this was proved when a doctor, James Carroll (1854–1907) of the USA, allowed himself to be bitten by an infected mosquito and died of the disease. The special nature of many tropical diseases was then established, by the old process of identifying the clinical disease and then searching for its cause, so that it might be prevented or a cure for it rationally sought.

Preventive medicine and a concern for the public health was a product of this century. Thomas Southwood Smith (1788–1861) was a Unitarian minister—an interesting comment on the relationships between religion and its practical action in social activity—who published *Philosophy of Health* in 1835. He helped found the Health of Towns Association in 1840, and he became a member of the General Board of Health, a new government department in the UK.

Edwin Chadwick (1800–1890) also was not a medical man, but after serious epidemics he was instrumental in founding a Sanitary Commission, in 1839. A Registration Act had been passed in 1838, which required that births, marriages and deaths should be registered, the first national attempt to gather vital statistics. By 1848 there came the first Public Health Act and under its provisions a General Board of Health was set up. The whole panoply of public health was then being formally organized, and its concerns have always been with the environment in prevention of disease, ensuring the provision of pure water and food, hygiene, sanitation and housing, and indeed preventing anything that can harm the health of individuals in the community. Medical Officers of Health were appointed by Liverpool and London, and the first in the metropolis was John Simon (1816–1904) who later moved to the General Board of Health, whose functions were taken over in 1917 by the new Ministry of Health. The United States and all other 'western' countries moved along the same lines, though with some organizational differences.

Interestingly, this general activity began before there was knowledge of bacteriology. It is not infrequent to find that empirical responses in medicine precede the scientific reasons for their efficacy. It seems as if something must be done to solve a problem using the best available though incomplete evidence, and that this action then stimulates others to find out whether the action has sound foundations.

Another general movement of the times was in nursing. This is another example of the effect of war and of military surgery on the general medical weal. Florence Nightingale (1820–1910) (*Figure 9.8*) during the Crimean War of 1854–57 took

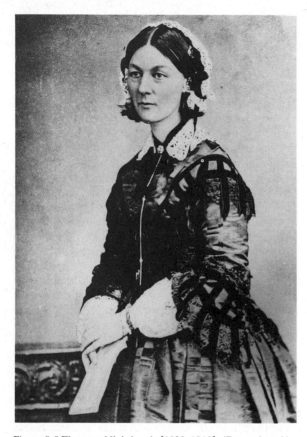

Figure 9.8 Florence Nightingale [1820–1910]. (Reproduced by courtesy of the Wellcome Institute Library, London)

nurses to the wards of the military hospital at Scutari, where she was appalled by the conditions in which the wounded were kept. She was an autocratic woman of iron will and imposed her ideas of nursing and medical care on those in authority and on her nurses. She had friends in the high place of the Cabinet. Through an endless stream of correspondence and personal overwhelming contacts she determined to improve nursing education and care whenever and wherever she could. It can only be said that she succeeded mightily, in that every nurse, every patient, every hospital design, the organization of medical and nursing services everywhere, owe something to her indomitable spirit. Like that other 'revolutionary', Charles Darwin, she achieved this partly through retreating from active affairs into a mysterious illness which kept her out of personal controversy, but did not prevent her voluminous correspondence influencing others to do her bidding and carry out her wishes. On her return from the Crimea she established the first School of Nursing in the world at St. Thomas's Hospital in London. From there her trained nurses went to all parts of the world, carrying her mission with them.

Hers was an incredible achievement. She founded a skilled profession, essential to the progress of medicine, out of what was then most unpromising material. Before her time those who nursed the sick were often ignorant, dirty, unprincipled, uneducated and without standards of any reasonable kind, with very few exceptions. She converted this rabble into the disciplined, caring, compassionate, educated force now expected and found everywhere in the civilized world.

Another movement, in the entry of women into the medical profession, began in 1849 when Elizabeth Blackwell (1821–1910), an Englishwoman, obtained a degree in New York.

The following year the Women's Medical College was started in Pennsylvania, and this was reserved purely for women. Prior to this time entry to medicine (with the thirteenth-century exception of Salerno, and perhaps some others) was restricted to men. The sometimes appalling sights of practice were deemed unsuitable for the tender susceptibilities of women, and it was thought that their modesty might be affronted in the intimate physical examination of patients. In England Elizabeth Garrett (1836–1917) qualified through the Society of Apothecaries' examination. The General Medical Council at first refused to register her, but later relented. Sophia Jex-Blake (1840–1913) with a few others managed to persuade the authorities in Edinburgh to accept them as students and to give them degrees, and when she qualified in 1876 the GMC had accepted that women should be admitted to the Medical Register. It was she and Elizabeth Garrett Anderson, with help from enlightened men, who founded the London School of Medicine in 1874 and this quickly became associated with the new Royal Free Hospital, where the women could obtain clinical training. The first battles for equality with men in medicine had been won, though there were still many to be fought, and even now, more than 130 years later, complete equality cannot be said to have been fully established.

This seething ferment of social, industrial, commercial, military, economic, scientific and medical forces demanded changes in the organization of medicine, just as in nursing. The ragged systems by which medical practitioners could qualify had to be brought into some sort of order. The usual way to qualify as a medical or surgical practitioner was to serve an apprenticeship, which was quite unstructured, and then to set up in practice either with or without passing some sort of examination by the Apothecaries, or Royal Colleges of Surgeons or Physicians. These examinations, by present standards, were perfunctory. The Physicians in particular had a long-established monopoly in London which allowed only those who held their licence to practise in the metropolis and its immediate surrounds. They also granted extra-licences for those practising elsewhere. Yet in the early years of the nineteenth century their examinations were conducted orally in Latin and demanded only some exposition of the classical Greek and Latin medical authors, so little recent knowledge was demanded. Only graduates of the universities of Oxford and Cambridge were permitted to take the examination, and in those ancient places the candidates studied the classics, botany and materia medica and had virtually no contact with patients. The Surgeons at least demanded an apprenticeship and some knowledge of anatomy, while the Apothecaries had to know something in practice with a master about medical therapeutics. It is of some importance that it was this century that determined the divisions of the profession into physicians, surgeons and general practitioners which have persisted in Britain. This separation was imposed in London, mainly, by the ways of entry to the profession as just outlined.

Moreover, London and other metropolitan cities had specialist hospitals founded during the nineteenth century, and round the turn of the century. Over the decades they have come in obstetrics, diseases of women, for children, for ophthalmology, for diseases of the ear, nose and throat, for skin diseases and dentistry, and later still for orthopaedics. And for long there have been hospitals for nervous diseases and for chest diseases. They are interesting since they demonstrate a reaction to the increasing knowledge of their times, and also that specialists often have to escape from a too pervading influence of the general physicians and surgeons. Those nearly always believe at first that there is nothing in a new specialty with which they cannot deal. The specialists can only escape this attitude by moving away, until the specialty is firmly established. Then there is often a move back into the general hospitals to give some representation of each special discipline. This has happened with most of the subjects mentioned above. Specialists now find that their specialty cannot be practised in isolation, since all medicine and surgery has become a matter for teamwork. Each specialty needs all the others close by, and this has become the late twentieth century response to increasing specialization. It explains why so many special hospitals are having to close. They are unable to give a full range of care, which now can be done only by grouping all specialties under one roof.

Clearly this nineteenth century system of the control of medicine was not enough. There were concerns about it in the profession and in the educated public at large. There were several attempts to get Acts through Parliament to have things changed. Finally, in 1858 the first Medical Act was passed. This set up the General Medical Council which was to regulate entry to the profession by the establishment of a Medical Register. This was to enable the public to distinguish between those with suitable qualifications to practise medicine and those who did not. This is still its purpose. This meant that the Council (GMC) had to decide what a doctor at qualification should be expected to know, and this led to the GMC having the power to inspect institutions where medical education was given and to approve or disapprove them and the examinations they made of their students. It was a mechanism for imposing standards through the supervision of the whole educational process that produced doctors.

By 1867 the GMC had decided what a modern doctor must know before being admitted to the Register. The curriculum was to be of descriptive anatomy, general anatomy, physiology, chemistry, materia medica, practical pharmacy, medicine, surgery, midwifery and forensic medicine. The list is now interesting for showing what was then deemed important by the medical establishment. The basic sciences of anatomy and physiology are there and so are the major disciplines of medicine, surgery and midwifery. Legal duties are especially included under forensic medicine, and the rest is about medical therapy, which from our day shows a rather pathetic faith in its efficacy. Pathology, bacteriology, psychiatry and public health are missing . Nevertheless it was a start and it helped to ensure that all doctors should have a certain basic knowledge which ought to equip them to help their patients.

These early and subsequent efforts to control, improve and enhance the educational standards of the medical profession have undoubtedly had a beneficial effect in the service of patients. More important perhaps is the underlying idea that the profession as a whole owes a duty to the public as a whole and that the doctors must demonstrate to the public that they are discharging those duties satisfactorily. It demonstrates very forcibly that medicine is an important arm of society's endeavours. The public, through governmental agencies, has rights over the practice of medicine and, in dialogue with the public, the medical profession has duties to the society it serves. This has always been true, at least in part, but in the

GMC and its accountability to the Privy Council these rights and duties received formal, though muted, expression. It will be seen that in the second half of the twentieth century the dialogue and relationships between public and profession have sharpened considerably. The pattern of control of medical education by the GMC has been emulated in various ways nearly everywhere in the world.

The nineteenth century is an amazing one to contemplate now. Its high point for intellectual development, from which ultimately everything else flows, was Darwin and all he stood for. He brought a new way of thinking about biological material; human, animal and plant. It has been emphasized in this chapter that he was not alone. The whole intellectual climate was moving in this direction. Conceptually the world became a different place after those mid-Victorian times. There was established a continuity from physical, geological and chemical materials to those of biology, including Man. The awkward leap to include psychology in this hierarchy was not made with any confidence, nor was it easy to see the place of God in the new scheme of things. The problems are still with us. Fuelling all was a certainty in the right order of things as they were socially and a sureness of stability. This gave confidence in the future and a belief that the mind of Man, through science in particular, was capable of continuing conquest of nature in technology and understanding.

It is easy to detect in retrospect the seeds of destruction of this generally complacent attitude. This climate of opinion generated the beginnings of cellular pathology and bacteriology to help in the delineation, classification and understanding of disease. Anaesthesia began the conquest of pain, and all these liberated surgery and obstetrics to bring about wonders never before envisaged. The prevention of disease became a real possibility because its nature was now more completely understood, mainly in infections which were the major killers and producers of illness then. This helped to funnel endeavours into the improvement of the public health, where government aid and intervention were obviously necessary. This caused critical examination of the role of the doctors, who along with the nurses were made to become professions with educational standards required to match the expectations of the public. It was an age too in which specialization began and many specialist hospitals were founded. The polymaths of medicine could no longer entirely hold their own against anatomists, physiologists, chemists, physicists, bacteriologists, pathologists and others, while even the clinical practitioners were split into physicians, surgeons (some specializing) and apothecaries, with each seldom trespassing on the preserves of the other. The changes wrought in so many human enterprises in Darwin's century have their repercussions still.

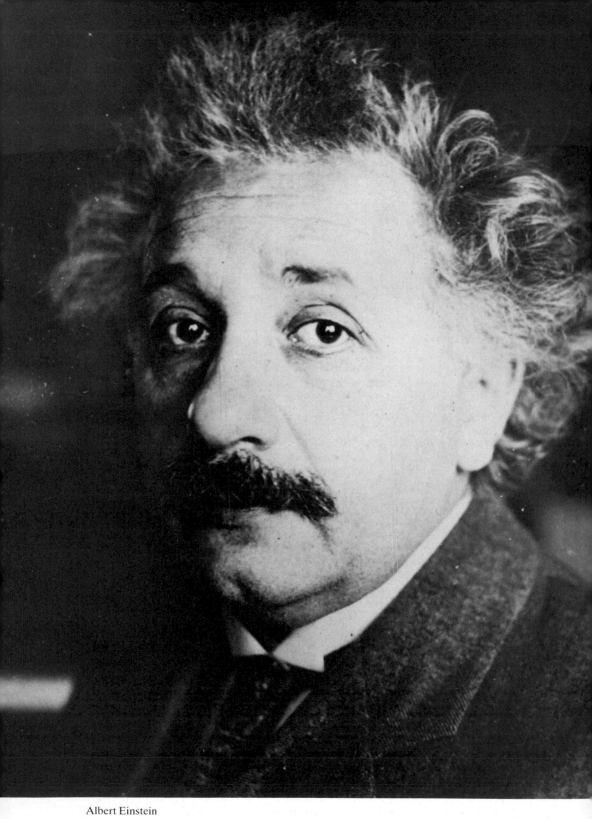

Albert Einstein

Chapter 10

Specialization (Twentieth century)

The nineteenth century generated enormous power in Europe. This was manifest in science and technology, which flourished within the Industrial Revolution. There was intellectual power supplemented and complemented by economic, financial, military and naval power. The rest of the world could not withstand it, so that European culture was established virtually all over the globe. It reached America, both north and south, Australia, New Zealand, Africa and many parts of the near and far East. Some of it was imposed by conquest and colonialism. Some of the culture was adopted and adapted by countries with which Europeans came in contact as the only defence against it. The older cultures elsewhere could not cope with overwhelming European ideologies, and so had to take on some of their colour in order to preserve something for themselves and their own way of life. This type of reaction to pressure was more pervasive, more subtle and undermining in the long run than colonialism and conquest. These last two forces have tended to retreat in the twentieth century as the oppressed have thrown off the foreign oppressors, yet much of the alien culture has remained. Ultimately, the only forces that can oppose ideas are other ideas, which seem acceptable to a particular culture at the time. Physical force, however exerted, cannot stamp out ideas, which are ultimately the generators of action. It is sad that thoroughgoing men of action have not learned this lesson, for if they did (which they will not) much of war and violence would be seen to be in the long term ineffective and unproductive.

Because of this near-ubiquity of European culture, advances in western-type science and medicine now come from all over the world. No country has a monopoly of scientific and technological discovery, so articles and books pour off the presses to be almost instantly available everywhere. These massive increases in communication and information have created scientific, technological and medical communities transcending many national boundaries. This has been much helped by the nearly universal use by science of the language of English, and to a lesser extent of French and German, in the literature of interest to scientists, technologists, engineers and doctors. The spread of English as a common language is essentially left over from colonialism, which for these purposes must include the United States of America. It is that country which is now at the forefront of advance in so much of science and technology. This is yet another example of the way in which these disciplines are associated with economic and military power and an ideology (however imperfect) that allows freedom of expression and pursuit of

117

knowledge with little hindrance. Russia could perhaps vie with the USA in intellectual achievement, but its economy is still weak, and its ideology constrains its individualists and potential intellectual leaders. The same is true of China and of Islam.

It is of more than passing interest to see how the major centres of medical progress have moved from Mesopotamia to Ionia, to Greece, Alexandria, Rome, northern Italy, northern Europe and onwards to north America. Always this progress has been part of a general growth of power—in industry, commerce, economy and finance, in military and naval affairs, and in those of the intellect. Medical progress is closely dependent on general progress. Those engaged too closely in intellectual matters, such as medicine, often seem to be quite unaware of this substrate which conditions everything they do. It has a message for the future in that medical advances will go mainly to those countries making economic progress. It is interesting to speculate where these will be when and if the USA should decline.

During the nineteenth and twentieth centuries world population continued to increase and was accompanied everywhere by a drift of people to the towns and cities, where industries and commerce provided employment. Rural populations relatively diminished and evidence shows that they tended to suffer from different diseases than those of their city cousins. In 1801 the population of the United Kingdom was about 12 million, by 1901 about 38 million and in 1981 about 56 million. London's population in 1840 was about 2 million and in 1981 was about 6.7 million. This sort of change went on world-wide. Moreover, there was much movement by migration. One estimate is that between 1840 and 1930 about 50 million people left Europe for other countries abroad. They too carried European ideologies with them. Their descendants still largely hold to European values, modified only in small measure by the differences of place and the passage of time.

Astonishingly it has to be reckoned that food supply, based in agricultural production, kept pace with this increasing number of mouths to feed, for world population rose 2–3 times in the nineteenth century and the process continues. It causes great anxiety because of the threats of over-population, which could only be redressed on present thinking by war, famine, disease or birth control. Few have seriously contemplated death control by killing off the aged or allowing them to die, for some of the population increase is occasioned by people living longer than formerly. This too is interesting since rising longevity antedates what might be looked on as major medical advances, especially those curing infections that have until recently been the major killers.

If better health can be measured by the increasing numbers of the elderly, then it seems to be more dependent on non-specific factors such as housing, clothing, warmth, sanitation, hygiene, pure food and water, control of epidemics and similar public health measures, than on specific curative medical advances. These have of course contributed by improved obstetrics, by vaccination, immunization and by antibiotics, and no doubt in many other ways. Nevertheless these contributions are small when compared with the effects of non-specific factors. No humanitarian would wish for war, famine and disease to continue unchecked, therefore much effort has been directed to perfecting contraception and abortion to control births.

There are effective and relatively safe techniques for this now, but the real problem is how to persuade sufficient numbers of people to use them. In other words it is cultural and other resistance to their use that must be overcome. Of course acceptance of birth control can be encouraged by government action, such as high taxation for those with families deemed to be too large, and other penalties and inducements can be legislated for, though not normally in fully democratic societies. All these methods of social policy and its enforcement and encouragement have been used in various countries, for population size is important economically and militarily. In the past the economy and armed force were entirely dependent on muscular power and the numbers of people pressed into service, if not servitude. Now, with other sources of energy available through machines of all kinds, there is less need for direct human production and the worry extends to the probability that too many people will generate too much demand and consume too many resources and goods. Such political and economic factors are complex and hard to define closely.

But one thing begins to stand out clearly from the experience of some advanced countries, and that is that when living standards are high then couples begin to limit their family sizes voluntarily. This is because they have other expectations in the ownership of consumer durables such as cars, cookers, television sets and so forth, and seem willing to cut down on numbers of children in order to have other things and to own more material goods. Cultural acceptance of birth control is apparently dependent on rising living standards and literacy. However, these may not be rapidly attainable unless combined with some reduction of the rate of rise of consumer demand by birth control. Several policies must be pursued concurrently. Among these must be the increase of agricultural production.

The matter of migration calls attention once more to transport. In the early years of the twentieth century this was still by horse, by railway and by steamship. By 1910 the Wright brothers had flown their first aeroplane and Zeppelin had produced an airship. No one now needs reminding of the immense progress made in air travel since then. Present airline services straddle the world, giving greater chances for more and more people to see each other in their home countries and to communicate with them. This communication has been formalized in medical and scientific conferences, small and large, everywhere. The exchange of information has been speeded up enormously. The telephone, radio and television and artificial satellites have added their vast quota to the communication and information explosion, as have newspapers and journals. Medical journals are now to be numbered in thousands published each year, mirroring the growth in specialization. Indeed so specialized have many periodicals and articles become that they are intelligible only to the very few mostly concerned with the particular discipline. The generalist has become submerged in the sea of specialization.

For the practice of medicine the response to the flood of knowledge and information has had to be teamwork. It is only in the simplest diseases that a single doctor is adequate for the care of a patient. Anything slightly complex requires the help of many others. There are now about 50–60 specialties in medicine, depending on how they are classified. A doctor can therefore spend a lifetime in the practice of a specialty and not fully comprehend it. There is now no way in which a doctor can encompass all the specialties. For comprehensive care of a patient in the western world a team of specialists is requisite. This has some faint reflection in papers written for medical journals. Increasingly these now have many authors, whereas single authorship was the rule at the turn of the century. Moreover, there were then few references to anyone else's work. Now each paper usually carries a long list of other papers, articles and books to be consulted by the reader for him to be fully informed of the subject under consideration.

Knowledge is then fragmented and dispersed, and often hard to retrieve when it is needed. The problem has not yet been solved, though computer technology of several different kinds may help to give a solution. The question is posed not only for medicine. It is pertinent to every sphere of knowledge. There may come some hope of an answer too from the fact that knowledge not only accumulates, it becomes obsolete. This is attested by every ancient library, where volume after volume gathers dust and is consulted by nobody because its messages have been superseded and they no longer have relevance to the problems of today. They were problems but are so no more. The advance of today becomes the commonplace of tomorrow, and it may be hard to understand why our ancestors found so much difficulty. Perhaps the twentieth century needs an all-embracing theory to unify the vast numbers of diverse observations in the natural sciences and particularly in biology and medicine, such as Newton and Darwin gave in their own times. The disparate elements of knowledge in their times must have looked just as chaotic to our forebears as ours do now to us. The great theories do let in the light and bring some order and sense out of the chaos. It might have been hoped that such unification would come in the twentieth century out of physics, and perhaps at the hands of Albert Einstein (1879–1955), but his theories of relativity seem not to have been incorporated into general workaday science, which in subjects outside physics is often still in the age of Newton.

Apart from the social upheavals consequent on population growth and movement the western world (that of European culture and descent) was convulsed by the two wars of 1914–18 and 1939–45. The second was more global than the first, and nearly the whole world was sucked into it directly or indirectly. For science, technology, engineering and medicine there were gains from war, as will emerge later. The advances in transport, communication, flight, blood transfusion, surgery, preventive medicine, anaesthesia, antibiotics and biophysics would no doubt have come sooner or later, but they were enormously accelerated in introduction by the demands of warfare. War gives a fillip to all forms of technological and scientific progress. There is a concerted effort to prosecute the task in hand—the defeat of the enemy—and money pours into research and development without stint. The results are not only immediate but they also have spin-offs into many peacetime endeavours, including medicine, though the pace slows down as effort and money is dissipated in myriad objectives of policy. The single end to which war is bent dissolves into an immense variety of ends, like a torrential river in a narrow canyon breaks up into the rivulets of a delta.

The century opened with an intellectual bang, made by Max Planck (1858–1947), who in 1900 produced the beginnings of the quantum theory. Energy thereafter, following many subsequent researches, has been seen as being dispensed in discrete packets (quanta) and not as a continuous stream, as had been formerly believed. This began a new train of thought in the relationships between matter and energy. Einstein took the concept further in his Special Theory of Relativity in 1905 and his General Theory in 1916. Put at its very simplest this imported time into the nature of things and where space and time had been thought of as separate entities they were now combined in a space–time continuum. The amateur onlooker can only marvel at the soaring flights of intellect of such a man. It is certain that the present tyro cannot possibly understand, and especially when it all seems to be epitomized in the simple formula $E=mc^2$, where E=energy, m=mass and c=the velocity of light!

One feels that the concept should be seminal, but so far it has not been in biology and medicine. If it were, who knows where it might lead? At least it implies an interconvertibility of mass and energy, and it also puts the observer in the scene in such a way that he may influence results obtained by present scientific experiment. This has been known at a simpler level in medicine, where the interactions of doctor and patient in consultation influence the situation such that the observer cannot be kept out of the experiment, but it seems that the same may be true of experiments with matter too. The consequences could be, possibly should be, of great importance. The old philosophy of subject and object and all that goes with it might be entirely superseded. There may not, in fact, be a material world 'out there' to be investigated as if it were totally independent of the observer. It may be a quite artificial division not in accord with reality. Subject and object may be a continuum, just as is space–time.

The further developments in physics and chemistry concerned the structure of the atom. The X-rays of Röntgen allowed for the investigation of atoms and crystals. The first was done by Ernest Rutherford (1871–1937) and Niels Bohr (1885–1962) and the second by Sir William Bragg (1862–1942) and his son Sir Lawrence (1890–1971). The Rutherford–Bohr atom was shown to have a nucleus, made up (as shown by subsequent researches) of a variety of mainly positively charged particles, and of shells of circulating electrons. Certain atoms containing 2, 8, 18 or 32 electrons were essentially stable, whereas those with intermediate numbers had apparent excesses or deficiencies of electrons in their outer shells. When one with an excess met one with a deficiency the extra electrons fitted into the spheres where there was deficiency and a chemical union resulted. The demonstration immediately made sense of chemical interactions and of the periodic table of Dimitry Ivanovich Mendeleev (1834–1907), a Russian, who had shown that all elements could be arranged in a series according to their atomic number, so that there were 92 elements.

The details are unnecessary here, but the concepts changed the nature of understanding of atomic and molecular structure, and by extension into biology and medicine have led to fuller knowledge of the whole of cellular physiology and pathology as in membranes, cytoplasm and nuclei, and in the biochemistry of enzymes, proteins and nucleic acids which function because of their shapes. The structure of molecules has led to pharmacologists being able, at least partially, to produce molecules of configurations that may be effective in curing or alleviating disease.

Another discovery was that by Pierre (1859–1906) and Marie (1867–1934) Curie of radium, and ultimately this has led on to the whole therapeutic system of radiotherapy. But in some ways more important was their discovery of plutonium and other substances which in radioactive decay were transformed into other substances, ending up with lead. Similarly, it was found later that atoms bombarded with an electron beam may give off high-speed particles and be transformed into some other substance. The immutability of matter as a concept has now gone for good. It is a seething mass of positively and negatively charged particles, for ever combining and recombining, and giving off particles and waves in quanta. Except with the inward eye of the advanced physicist it seems impossible to translate this in imagination to the world that we seem to know. The basis of our material world would appear to be made up of particles and waves and fields of force and even these dissolve into one another. Yet there must be something of importance lurking in these hard-to-grasp truths, for they are at the base of biochemistry, biophysics, electronics and much medical technology now in everyday use.

The pragmatic effects of these advances in physical understanding are there to be seen. Regrettably too there have been effects in the production of atomic and hydrogen and neutron bombs, but as an offshoot there has also been nuclear energy, which may yet with other sources help to solve the predicted forthcoming energy crisis if only the older fuels are used.

These researches in physics have had profound effects in medicine. The most obvious is in diagnostic and therapeutic radiology. The treatment of cancer in the early years of the century had to be surgical, for there was no other tool. Then it was realized that X-rays and gamma rays altered the functions of living cells, and the more rapidly these reproduce, as in cancer, the greater the effect in killing them. A new dimension was then added to treatment, and although deep-ray therapy has not been universally successful in all types of cancer there have been many valuable successes. However, the passage of time has shown that there can be unpleasant side-effects of X-ray therapy (even the inducing of cancer), both to the individual treated and to the genes of their children. These risks have been diminished somewhat by refining techniques and by different physical means of producing therapeutic rays, but they have not been banished, though radiotherapy may gradually be superseded by chemical cancer chemotherapy.

Diagnostic radiology has been in the forefront of imaging techniques, so that pictures of the interior of the body may be obtained. Everyone knows of these in the diagnosis of fractures of bones, and in diseases of the lungs. Contrast media of chemical compounds introduced into the body cavities heighten the value of these diagnostic radiographs; taken by mouth or injected into the bloodstream or a cavity, contrast media mean that virtually every system of the body may be displayed pictorially, though often somewhat imperfectly. But physics has come to the rescue again by the understanding it has given of isotopes and of the structure of the atom in nuclear magnetic resonance. Isotopes are small quantities of normally occurring biological atoms which give off waves of radiation. When injected the molecules in which these isotopes are incorporated are treated by body metabolism in the same way as the natural substances. Where they get to can be visualized by their radioactivity. Many organs concentrate substances differentially, the most obvious one being the thyroid gland and iodine, but now there are many others. And some tumours do the same, so that they may be 'seen' indirectly distinct from the normal structures.

Nuclear magnetic resonance uses magnetic fields and radio waves to give evidence of certain molecules, and these two can be made by physical means to produce an image for viewing. This promises to be a most valuable diagnostic tool for it can give biochemical evidence of what is happening in various parts of the body without harm and without invasion of any kind. It may in fact partially displace computerized axial tomography (CAT) scanning from its present (1984) position. This scanning is a superb example of the combining of physics, mechanical engineering and electronic engineering with anatomy, pathology and radiology. An X-ray beam is made to rotate round the body and from the many separate pictures a single composite picture is built up by computer technology. The display is of a narrow transverse section of the body. For decades anatomists have taught cross-sectional anatomy, and no serious use could be found for it. This advance in body-imaging has made it into a useful discipline. Much apparently esoteric work comes into its own when technology can combine it with something else to make it of practical use. On the other hand, much research undoubtedly quite properly goes into limbo, but the problem is that no one can foresee which will find its place in practice and which will disappear. For sensible people this is the major argument for supporting fundamental research whose useable outcome cannot be predicted. Rutherford and Bohr were not looking for applications of their work on the atom, but these have come rapidly in war and in peace. Politicians have been glad of them in different ways, while often deploring unnecessary, impractical and wasteful scientific research, or paying it only marginal attention.

In like fashion it would not at first have been possible to forecast that the radar waves of Robert Watson-Watt (1892–1973), discovered about 1935, would be used not only for finding ships and aeroplanes, but also in the development of ultrasound for diagnosis in medicine and particularly at first by Ian Donald (1910–) of Glasgow in obstetrics. Developments in optical physics and engineering technology have produced instruments allowing the projection of light along flexible fibre-optic rods, so that an observer can look directly into cavities and the lumina of tubes. Another contribution of physics to medicine has been the electron microscope (*Figure 10.1*). With its very short wavelengths and other physical technology the interior structure of cells and their membranes has been explored, beyond earlier belief. Some large molecules have actually been seen. These ultra-structural studies have dovetailed with genetics and molecular biology in all their present ramifications. The various specialties are now impossible to review as if they were separate from one another. They dissolve into one another and have no real boundaries between them. There is total continuity from physics to chemistry, to biology and medicine. Simple concepts cannot cope with this complexity.

There is no need here to dwell on the development of chemistry in isolation from biochemistry, physiology, genetics, pharmacology and nutrition. Suffice it to say that the physical and chemical techniques have been refined and improved, so that biological and medical investigations have been suggested, and chemists have had problems put to them for solution because biologists and doctors needed them. The nexus of science is now so vast that in tracing interactions of its various parts in recent history almost any path can be taken through the network and in some degree it will be true. The Nobel Prizes in physics, chemistry and physiology–medicine, instituted in 1901, pick out some of the highlights of progress, but looking through the lists of winners it often seems impossible to categorize their work into one or other of these headings. Crystallography, for instance, previously mentioned, is both physical and chemical. Spectroscopy—in which emissions and absorptions of light by various substances, so that chemical substances, often of enormous complexity, may be analysed and quantitatively measured—is physical and chemical. Radioimmunoassay uses physical methods and biological ones to measure quantities of complex molecules. And there are other varieties of immunochemistry in which animals and people may be used to raise antibodies to materials, and antigen–antibody reactions can be measured.

There is no foreseeable end to the ingenuity in which physical, chemical and biological techniques can be combined and recombined to give information of value in all these subjects. They have given great service in medicine, both in understanding and in practice.

Anatomy in the twentieth century has passed beyond discoveries in macroscopic, topographical morphology. Its concerns have moved into neuroanatomy, embryology, cellular biology and immunology, as well as anthropology, zoology, ecology, behaviour and human palaeontology. Apart from its original core of topographical anatomy it is scarcely recognizable as a distinct subject, since it has shaded off into many realms of biology, particularly cellular. Its ancient core

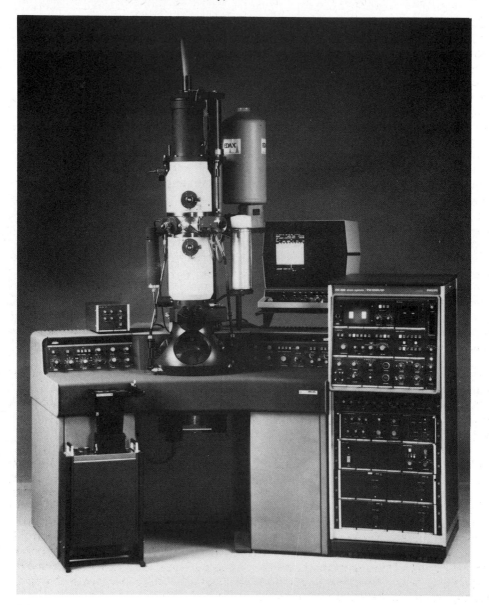

Figure 10.1 Electron microscope

remains an essential basis for the practice of medicine, and especially surgery and obstetrics, and also of the various forms of imaging techniques, using radiation, electromagnetic and other waves. This change in the nature of the discipline has brought problems in medical education. The organization of this was laid down from Renaissance and later times and has tended to persist, perhaps taking too little notice of changes that have occurred, and not only in anatomy.

Physiology likewise has become difficult to disentangle conceptually from medicine, pathology, physics and chemistry, cellular biology and pharmacology. The textbooks forever call on techniques, concepts and investigations in these various fields, on which physiology draws and to which it adds its own dimensions. This real indivisibility of all the sciences, especially in their relationships with the practice of medicine, needs constant reiteration. The divisions and categorizations are conceptual for ease of thought and contemplation. They are not real.

In 1902 Ernest Henry Starling (1866–1927), with William Bayliss (1860–1924) in London, isolated secretin from the duodenum and showed that it passed in the bloodstream to the pancreas, causing that organ to discharge digestive enzymes into the gut. Two years later Starling named such substances 'hormones', meaning that they stir up or excite the target organs on which they have their effects. This began the whole series of investigations into endocrine glands, which secrete their substances entirely into the bloodstream, in contrast with the exocrine glands which use a duct to convey their secretions on to a surface. The subject of endocrinology has expanded so greatly that some physicans devote themselves entirely to it, in its physiological and pathological manifestations, while basic scientists may work for a lifetime in only one aspect of its subdivisions. More than this, endocrinology has altered concepts of bodily functions and communications between organs, tissues and cells. Fast responses to stimuli, arising within or outside the body, come from nerve and muscle. But these can only come about because of the slower responses mediated in large measure by the endocrine system. The molecules of the many hormones carry messages to stimulate activity of their effector organs. They are major contributors to the maintenance of the relative constancy of the internal environment, as first enunciated by Claude Bernard. It is not surprising to find that Starling made many contributions to understanding of this in matters of fluid balance and in control mechanisms of the heart.

But the major interest lies in the recognition that the fast responses that are observed in our everyday lives are based on a stable continuum of metabolism, to which much of the bodily economy is devoted.

Pursuing the same general theme in a different way was Charles Sherrington (1857–1952) (*Figure 10.2*), who produced *The Integrative Action of the Nervous System* in 1906. This gathered together the thoughts on the actions of the spinal cord and brain that have dominated researches and insight since. He noted the sensory receptors as those responding to stimuli coming from outside the body (exteroceptive), those coming from within (interoceptive) and those arising in the joints and muscles (proprioceptive). The stream of impulses reaching the central nervous system have to be recognized, assembled, and put into some sort of order by integration. Then appropriate reactions can be initiated, and these cover the responses of which an animal or person is capable—all bodily movements, sleeping, eating, excretion, secretion and metabolism.

The book has coloured all subsequent thought about the nervous system. With Edgar Adrian (1889–1977), Sherrington won the Nobel Prize in 1932 for work on the nerve impulse. This brought in the important concept that impulses come in discrete packets, the intensity of the stimulus being translated into the number and frequency of the impulses generated. Moreover, there is a threshold stimulus, meaning that a subliminal one fails to excite an impulse but that a liminal one triggers off the impulse in an 'all-or-none' reaction. Nerve impulses come off in packets all of the same size, just as quanta do. The intensity of the energy is measured by the numbers of quanta, not by their individual sizes, which are all the same. The other important feature of this work was that the impulse was shown to

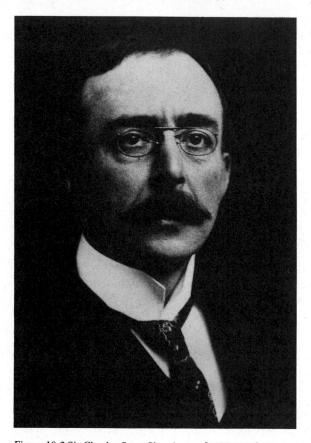

Figure 10.2 Sir Charles Scott Sherrington [1857–1952]. (Reproduced by courtesy of the Wellcome Institute Library, London)

be electrophysicochemical in nature. The highest reaches of biological evolution, in the central nervous system, are therefore apparently to be explained in these more basic terms. This concept has now guided biological and medical science over several decades. In practice it has brought enormous gains, yet philosophically it has posed problems of body–mind relationships and psychosocial interactions. Adrian himself was well aware of this and wrote on the theme in *The Basis of Sensation* in 1927.

In about 1909 Henry Dale (1875–1968) worked on the hormone pituitrin, extracted from the posterior lobe of the pituitary gland deep inside the skull, and found that it had actions on blood vessels in controlling the blood pressure and on causing contractions of the uterus. He also pushed forward researches into the transmission of nerve impulses in the central nervous system when he demonstrated that at the synapse between the axon (the process of a nerve cell which conveys impulses in one direction only) and the cell body of another nerve cell the impulse is conveyed by the chemical substance acetylcholine. This meant that the electrophysicochemical impulses released a chemical, which in its turn produced other electrophysicochemical changes in the next nerve cell in the chain. Since the cells are in contact though separate from each other, the acetylcholine must induce changes in the cell membrane. Nowadays much research is devoted to the properties of cell membranes which is a major branch of cell biology. Acetylcholine has many other functions outside the nervous system, and it is also used (though not so much as formerly) pharmacologically. Dale's work was therefore on the boundaries of physiology, biochemistry and pharmacology, and it was recognized when with his collaborator Otto Loewi (1873–1961)—a German—they were awarded the Nobel Prize in 1936. Their original discovery was made in 1914.

John Scott Haldane (1860–1936) elucidated much in the physiology of respiration. In 1905 he found that breathing was regulated greatly by the tension of carbon dioxide in the blood, and he introduced a simple measurement for the amount of haemoglobin circulating. This measurement has become routine in clinical medicine for part of the diagnosis of anaemia. Haldane was interested in the physiological adaptations to high altitude, and for this purpose took an expedition to Pike's Peak in Colorado. Developments of this work have been essential for mountaineering, aviation and the space programme. His work on respiration in miners and on the deadly effects of carbon monoxide poisoning as well as those of other gases made their contributions to occupational medicine. In addition he investigated deep sea diving and brought in the method of slow decompression to prevent the bends, which have so sorely afflicted divers. Again the developments in underwater exploration and exploitation of the sea-bed owe much to pioneers like him.

In the USA in 1914 Edward Calvin Kendall (1886–1972) isolated the hormone, thyroxine, from the thyroid gland. A little later he found glutathione, so important in many aspects of cellular respiration. With Philip S. Hench (1896–1965) he isolated the hormones of the adrenal gland, for which they were awarded the Nobel Prize in 1950. This emphasized the enormous importance of steroid compounds in all aspects of metabolism. There are now scientists who devote their lives to only a small proportion of the known steroids, which have their uses in therapy for many acute and chronic diseases. These two men wrought a revolution in biological understanding and in medical practice, including surgery.

In Russia was Ivan Petrovich Pavlov (1849–1936), who received the Nobel Prize in 1904 in connection with work on the digestive system. He is more renowned now for his researches into conditioned reflexes which were prosecuted in the period from about 1898 to 1930. He showed that a dog salivating at the sight and smell of food may after an experimental period of conditioning by being shown a shape at the same time as seeing the food, be induced to salivate at the sight of the shape alone. This demonstrates an association of ideas in the mind (brain) of the dog, which normally would be dissociated. The dog has therefore learned. There are many now who may criticize the design and interpretation of these experiments, but Pavlov pointed the way towards investigation of the higher reaches of the nervous system, in the cortex and subcortical nuclei. His work interdigitated with that of Sherrington. Also he pointed towards a new way of looking at psychic phenomena, which has not entirely disappeared from psychological and psychiatric theory. Indeed operant conditioning as a means of psychological treatment is still much practised. Aversion therapy in which a formerly pleasant act is associated with (say) an unpleasant repeated electric shock is also used to rid the patient (client) of undesirable personal and anti-social habits and attitudes.

Understanding of the functions of the central nervous system has come also from myriad observations in the laboratory and clinically. Injuries of wartime with trauma of many kinds ablating parts of the brain and spinal cord, or severing fibre tracts in them, have given much insight and have suggested types of laboratory investigation to elucidate the clinical and post-mortem observations. Surgeons and physicians, too numerous to mention individually, have made lasting contributions in this way. Electron microscopy has added its quota in revealing large areas of the nervous system not previously seen, so adding further complexity to an already difficult subject. Computers too have suggested analogies for the way in which the brain might work, with excitation and inhibition, or positive and negative feedback, in immense variation. However, the previous analogy that the central nervous system worked like a vast telephone exchange has had to go by the board, and probably the analogy of the computer will go the same way. Conceptually the analogues may have temporary helpfulness, but the brain is neither a telephone exchange nor a simple computer. It has flights beyond these man-made machines which are not fully to be explained away in their terms, to whatever power the machines may be raised. There is much more to come yet, even though artificial intelligence has arrived in the form of electronic computers. Amazing though these are in what they can do it is easy to predict that as analogues for brain function they will, in their present form, go the way of the telephone exchange.

Hints about the development of endocrinology have already been given, but some further consideration is needed. Dale, for instance, found histamine in 1910. It is to be found almost everywhere in the body. It is not looked on as a hormone in the classic sense of Starling, but it has effects on cellular metabolism and on inflammatory reactions and in stimulating digestive processes in the stomach. So it is not a hormone produced by an identifiable endocrine gland but is produced in a wide variety of discrete tissues. The same is true of cyclic-AMP which is concerned with actions within the cells and in their membranes. In 1949 R. Kurzrock and C. C. Lieb discovered prostaglandins when they put seminal fluid into the uterine cavity and found that the uterus contracted. The substance causing this effect was thought to come from the male prostate gland, but later researches have found prostaglandins in every tissue, where they produce a variety of effects, and they have been characterized as a series of compounds and not just one. Similar discoveries have been made about the steroid or sterol compounds. Their chemistry has been unravelled and types of them are the main secretions of the adrenal glands, the ovaries and the testes. But in a bewildering variety they occur everywhere as cholesterol or one of its derivatives and play their parts in cellular metabolism.

A major step came in 1921 when Frederick Banting (1891–1941) and Charles H. Best (1899–1978) in Toronto discovered insulin in the islets of the pancreas. Deficiency of this hormone is the cause of diabetes. As a result of their work and that of John J. R. Macleod (1876–1935) who worked in London, Cleveland (Ohio) and Toronto, diabetes became more successfully treatable, and its worst effects could be staved off. It is the commonest of endocrine diseases, but since 1921 it has had many of its terrors, infirmities and premature deaths removed. Of course there have been many advances since in treatment and in understanding, but they all stem from this first discovery, for which Banting and Macleod received the Nobel Prize in 1923, a richly deserved honour for the good they wrought.

The century has seen intense investigations into the pituitary gland, the thyroid, pancreas, adrenals, ovaries and testes. The results have been deeper understanding of their functions and diseases and of their places in integration of the bodily economy. And to some degree their control and integration resides in the central nervous system. Adrenalin, for instance, is produced by some nerve endings and also by the medulla of the adrenal gland. It has major effects all over the body, but particularly on the cardiovascular system. Comparatively recently it has been found that parts of the central nervous system, particularly the hypothalamus at the base of the brain, produce hormones which act directly on the endocrine glands, and especially the pituitary, which is in part a controller of many other glands and their secretions. There is an astonishing interaction between them all. And rarely tumours arising in parts remote from a main gland may produce hormones which they would not have been expected to do. Again the boundaries are seen to be dissolving in a total integration which cannot be fully grasped in detail by anyone. Conceptually divisions have to be made for partial understanding, but the divisions are not real and they are all only elements in the edifice. There is no wonder that science, technology and medicine now require teams of specialists for the prosecution of their ends.

Sir Frederick Gowland Hopkins (1861–1947) ushered in a new era of biochemistry and nutrition. In 1901 he found the amino acid tryptophane, and later a series of amino acids which he showed could not be manufactured by the animal body but had to be provided in the diet. These he called essential amino acids, which in their combinations make up proteins. The sequence of a relatively few amino acids in long chains determines the properties and functions of the complex molecules of an almost infinite number of proteins. It is these that can be regarded as the very stuff of life, though this is much too simple a view. But they are one of life's major features, and without them no living creatures could exist. In lesser measure that is true of many other substances, but there is some part of truth in the belief that proteins are central to cellular function and so figure greatly in the subject of cell biology. Hopkins took the concept of essential food factors further in the finding of what are now known as vitamins. When he started his work it was thought that life could be sustained by protein, fat, carbohydrate, mineral salts and water. He showed, however, that when these were supplied to animals they still did not thrive. Something else, in small quantity, was needed. These were later characterized, and deficiency diseases were discovered, and the nature of night-blindness, some epithelial disorders, beri-beri, pellagra, scurvy and rickets became clearer. The discoveries came from all over the world. They have influenced agricultural policy in the growth of some crops rather than others, to help maintain adequate nutrition in poorer countries. They were of importance in food policies in the two major European wars. They even helped in the maintaining of good vision in night-fighter pilots.

Explorations and expeditions have had to take notice of the findings in nutrition. Some veterinary diseases have been found to be due to deficiencies of some minerals and other food factors in the soil. And more recently it has been shown that diseases in people may arise from lack of or excess of trace elements in the diet. Ultimately, all of these components of a diet are used in individual cellular function. The whole individual is the integrated sum of all his cells. Each of these has to have its membrane delineating it from its environment and yet exchanging with that enviroment, so that it may metabolize, respire, excrete, secrete and in some cases reproduce. All aspects of individual function are mirrored in cellular function. It is this that gives especial significance to modern cell biology.

A special fillip was given to the subject by the discovery of the double helix of desoxyribosenucleic acid (DNA) in the chromosomes of every cell nucleus. It is this that controls the function of the cell. Prior to the time of Francis Crick (1916–) and James Watson (1928–) with Maurice Wilkins (1916–), who elucidated the structure and composition of DNA and for which they received the Nobel Prize in 1962, there were many discrete observations in genetics and in chromosomal analysis and cellular function. These biologists were able to build on this progress in physics, chemistry, biochemistry, biophysics, clinical and animal genetics to produce their model of DNA and how it worked. The results have been amazing. The structure is of two chains of only four nucleic acids bound together in set patterns; but by arranging the acids in different sequences, different properties result.

The sequences determine, by their shapes, which amino acids shall be introduced, and in what order, into protein molecules. The sequence of amino acids in various proteins is therefore dependent on the sequences of nucleic acids in DNA. DNA is the template on which proteins are fashioned. This forms the basis of cellular function and of heredity. The general simplicity of this system when compared with the infinite complexity of living things is almost incredible. It is comparable with the work of Darwin in the insights it has given and continues to give. One special outcome of value for medicine has been in the genetic manipulation of bacteria to make them produce therapeutic substances of a complexity that even modern chemistry could not manufacture. After just over 20 years since the Nobel Prize was awarded it is still too early to judge the full significance of the discovery of the double helix and how it works. It has opened up tremendous vistas in terrain that is still being explored, and that brings fresh discoveries every day in theory and in practice. It is a key which unlocks many hitherto closed doors.

A new chapter in immunology came in 1901, when Karl Landsteiner (1868–1943) discovered the major blood groups of the ABO system. Some antigen–antibody reactions to bacteria and toxins were known, and Emil von Behring (1854–1917) received the first Nobel Prize in physiology and medicine in 1901, for his work with serum therapy mainly in the treatment of diphtheria. But Landsteiner demonstrated the reaction of the body to foreign tissue, and this has opened the way to blood transfusion, without which modern surgery and much of medicine would be impossible.

More important in general has been the whole idea of immune responses to another individual's organs and tissues, and even antibody reactions to his own tissues, as in the now widely recognized autoimmune diseases. This was shown in certain thyroid diseases when, for reasons unknown, a particular person might produce antibodies to his gland cells thus causing inflammation and destruction so that myxoedema (thyroid deficiency) resulted. Further developments in understanding of these responses is now such that organ transplantations have been made possible, as any reader of the general press will know. Because blood is fluid it is sometimes forgotten that in transfusion from one person to another a form of transplantation is being made, and just as with any similar operation there may be a host-versus-donor response in the production of antibodies which may cause undesirable side-effects and even death. Landsteiner's work showed that some blood groups are compatible with others when safe transfusion may be done. This is the reason for the cross-matching of the bloods of donor and recipient which is routine practice in hospitals nowadays before blood (and some other blood products) are transfused from one person to another. The concept has been enormously extended so that complex compatibility tests are done in the technique of tissue-typing when it is intended to transplant (say) the kidney, liver, heart or heart and lungs, from a donor to a new host. The technique depends on the recognition of whether a particular organ or tissue is or is not likely to cause a rejection reaction by the production of antibodies, so making the patient ill or causing his death. The underlying principles in blood transfusion and organ transplantation are similar.

In tissues such as the cornea of the eye it is fortunate that the foreign material does not excite a vigorous response in the recipient when transplanted, largely because there is a meagre vascular supply to the cornea and body responses are then at a minimum. Highly vascular organs, such as those of kidney and liver, must, however, be exposed to the bloodstream of the recipient. Recent work of course has led to discoveries of chemical substances that can be used to suppress and modify the response of the body to foreign transplanted material, so that transplant operations are increasingly successful, especially with kidneys.

The development of understanding and at least partial control of the immune responses of the body is a twentieth-century phenomenon. The early studies on humoral antibodies were at the end of the nineteenth century. Cellular responses to injury and infection were investigated by Elie Metchnikoff (1845–1916), a Russian who worked with Pasteur. He noted how white cells of the blood often engulfed bacteria in the process known as phagocytosis. Within the cells the bacteria often were killed, but sometimes they killed the cells. Almroth Wright (1861–1932) about 1903 at St. Mary's Hospital, London, investigated substances in the blood called opsonins which coat the white cells to help them phagocytose bacteria. Here were humoral and cellular responses acting together. A year earlier Alexis Carrel (1873–1944) in France was experimenting with transplanting organs and tissues and also with suturing severed blood vessels. He and Metchnikoff both ultimately received Nobel Prizes.

Much later still Macfarlane Burnet (1899–) of Australia and Peter Medawar (1915–) of England were awarded Nobel Prizes in 1960 for work on transplant antigens. Medawar, working with skin grafts in animals, demonstrated some of the mechanisms that cause rejection of donor grafts by hosts.

In some ways it is unfair to pick out these splendid achievements, for hundreds, perhaps thousands of other workers have made contributions that have filled in missing parts of a very complex jigsaw puzzle. And the story of immunity extends into other fields than transplantation, though that may be the most spectacular. Antibodies in the blood come in many different varieties. Some people are deficient in being able to withstand attacks from without or within, and several immunodeficiency diseases are now recognized. There may be over-reactions too between antibodies and antigens in disorders of hypersensitivity. Finally, the immune system is involved in the containment (or failure to contain) cancers and other tumours. For a long time it has been known that tumours may excite a reaction among the lymphocytes (small white cells of the blood) in a sort of inflammatory response. Now it is known that the lymphocytes are makers and bearers of antibodies and that they come from lymph glands, spleen, bone marrow and the thymus. The function of this gland has been hidden for centuries, but is now known to be a vital part of the immune system by the changes it brings about in lymphocytes.

These various immunological responses are of fundamental importance in biology. In very simple terms they identify for each individual what is self and what is not-self. They are the determinants of individual identity. This is based in heredity and in the genetic constitution. The genes in their arrangement within the chromosomes are unique for each individual. They control cell metabolism and function. There is a continuity from fertilization through to the fully fledged adult and on into old age and to death in which the individual is protecting himself and his personal identity from all the slings and arrows that beset him both from without and within. In constant change there is always the potential for things going wrong either within the body or induced by outside influence. To hold to personal identity and maintain personal integration is a struggle needed throughout life. Part of the armoury resides in the immune system, and just as in any conflict the arms may be turned against the invaders, or they may be too few for defence against attack, or they may be turned against the commonweal in a form of civil war.

Pathology, the scientific basis of clinical medicine, has particularly shown the tendency to specialization, so characteristic of the twentieth century. At the end of the last century a pathologist dealt with all branches. This is no longer possible and the discipline consists of morbid anatomy (histopathology), microbiology, haematology and chemical pathology. All are central to the practice of clinical medicine. They have helped to make diagnosis and treatment so much more exact than was possible in the early decades of the twentieth century. Clinical medicine was then very much a matter for the doctor at the bedside, and he depended on his own observations with little support felt to be needed from laboratory or radiology techniques. This has greatly changed so that the majority of patients in hospital and several in primary care facilities have special investigations made in order to check and make more precise the clinical diagnosis. Indeed some diseases can only be diagnosed in the laboratory or by some form of imaging or special viewing technique.

This brings with it the danger that clinical method at the bedside or in the clinic may be devalued, or even ignored entirely as of little importance. This tendency has to be and is being resisted. Laboratory tests are isolated phenomena within the total assessment of the patient and his illness. They are part of the evidence, not usually the whole of it. The corrective factors to be applied to that evidence have mainly to be derived from the clinical consultation. This is widely appreciated both by doctors who work in the clinical situation and by those in the laboratories. It is interesting that modern patients, when they do complain about their brushes with medicine, are most upset by insensitivity shown to them as individuals in the clinical environment. They take the technological backing of diagnosis and treatment for granted. Their concern is with relationships between themselves and those who care for them at the psychological and social levels. The clinical end of the spectrum of diagnosis and therapy requires constant and scrupulous care and attention. That which is out of sight of the patient in the laboratories and other diagnostic and therapeutic departments has to be left to the overview of the professionals. Their interface is with other professionals mainly, where misunderstandings might be expected to be at a minimum. It is the potential gulf between clinician and patient in their understanding of each other that needs special attention to communication, rapport and trust.

Histopathology is a part of morbid anatomy based on the macroscopic and microscopic examinations of organs, tissues and cells in the living and the dead. Originally the source of materials for examination came from autopsies. Now they come from specimens removed at surgical operation and by biopsies, which are done to remove small amounts of tissue specially for microscopic examination. There remains cultural opposition to post-mortem examinations, more especially in some parts of the world than others. However, autopsy is still necessary when the cause of death is unknown, and it is valuable as a check on the diagnosis made in life. Diagnoses have often to be made on inadequate evidence, or the evidence gained may be misread. To have the check of autopsy is a way of raising clinical standards, or at least maintaining them.

Despite some naïve beliefs to the contrary, medicine remains relatively crude and inexact clinically. Diagnosis and treatment require action in the minimum possible time. Everything may become clear in the course of a long time, but neither doctor nor patient can wait indefinitely, especially when the outcome of inaction may be death. Histopathological examination of operation and biopsy specimens is now routine. Insight into many diseases has come from advancing technology—in cutting specimens and preparing them for microscopic examination; in staining to make cellular structures visible; in optical techniques and the manufacture of microscopes and in electron microscopy. Theory and practice derive much from the advances in cellular biology, to which investigations into abnormal cells have made their contribution. Cytology (the examination of a few cells, appropriately stained, derived by scraping the surface of a tumour or normal tissue) has been added to the techniques of histopathology. Many have been involved in this development, but the name of George Nicholas Papanicolaou (1883–1962) is especially associated with it.

The subject of histopathology has made enormous strides during this century. It is established in every major hospital throughout the world. Modern medicine would be impossible to practise without it. It operates on the boundaries of physics, chemistry, biology and the clinical subjects. With thousands of workers involved it would be invidious to pick out a few names in a concise history. The subject is not dependent on the enterprise of a few. It is a superb example of the modern trends to make advances by a world-wide network, knowing no national barriers, and established by common interests, and with cellular pathologists aware of each other's researches through elaborate communication. It is a vast communal enterprise.

Microbiology too has made enormous strides since the days of Pasteur, Koch and others at the end of the nineteenth century. Hundreds, perhaps thousands, of disease-producing bacteria have been discovered and their natural history unravelled. In the first half of the twentieth century bacteriology helped to convert clinical medicine towards being a more exact science than ever before. Before Pasteur and his successors infective diseases had to be defined purely clinically from an assemblage of vague symptoms and physical signs, from the natural history of the disease and the use of the thermometer after it became established as a useful instrument to employ. Now Koch's postulates can be satisfied for an immense number of diseases caused by bacteria, so that diagnosis is often quite specific—one disease, one cause. (It has gone even further, as will be seen later, in that there is often a specific remedy for the infection.) Scientific bacteriology greatly added to understanding of immune mechanisms too. Antigens and antibodies were first defined in relation to bacterial infection, and then into blood-grouping, and there arose the science of serology—the investigation of reactions of many kinds taking place in serum. Octave Gengou (1875–1957) and Jules Jean Baptiste Vincent Bordet (1870–1961) of Belgium about 1900 discovered complement, the substance in serum that acts as a sort of intermediary to help in antigen–antibody reactions.

Just past the turn of the century there was much interest in syphilis. This is not surprising, for it is a chronic disorder affecting virtually every part of the body with dire effects. It was said to be the great mimic of many other diseases and therefore had to enter into the differential diagnosis for every patient. It had always to be on the list of possible diseases from which the patient was suffering. A serological test for syphilis was discovered by August von Wassermann (1866–1925), in Germany, so that there came a more or less specific test for the disease. It did not, however, give certainty in diagnosis, though it remained in vogue for several decades *faute de mieux*. Now there are more refined and accurate tests, though they are still based on the principles of the original Wassermann reaction (WR). And in 1905 Fritz Schaudinn (1871–1906) and Erich Hoffman (1868–1959) of Germany demonstrated microscopically the spirochaetal organism causing syphilis, and it could also be recognized in tissues by the use of a stain introduced by Constantin Levaditi (1874–1953) of Paris in 1905. However, the organisms cannot always be found though the search for them is diligent. Their serious effects remain even after they have disappeared from the scene, but by one method or another it is nearly always possible to be sure of the diagnosis nowadays (1984).

This shows a general principle that final diagnosis in many diseases depends on a multiplicity of approaches. The manifestations of disease are protean so that only rarely is it possible to point to a single diagnostically certain method.

Syphilis is only one example. The rest could become a long catalogue. Howard Taylor Ricketts (1871–1910) in America was on the trail of typhus, and his name became attached to a whole series of organisms (Rickettsiae). His work was around 1907. In 1923 George Frederick Dick (1881–1967) and Gladys Rowena Dick (1881–1963) of Belfast in Ireland discovered the streptococcus causing scarlet fever and a skin test to diagnose it. It was then a serious, maiming and killing disease. And the story has continued. At one time it almost seemed as if bacteriology were played out and that all worth while had been discovered, and that it had become a humdrum, routine series of investigations. This naïve, pessimistic view has been totally scouted, as anyone with an understanding of biological processes would have realized, even at the time of doubt. New diseases and new bacteria are discovered and reported on every few weeks (e.g. Lassa fever, Legionnaire's disease). The deep realization of the fundamental plasticity of all forms of life has been fostered by understanding bacterial behaviour. Bacteria formerly causing acute serious illness have become attenuated. Others, known of old or newly discovered, almost suddenly become virulent. Some escape the effects of antibiotics and other substances to which they had once been susceptible. Some change their genetic constitutions and some even occasionally reproduce in an almost sexual fashion. Some can be manipulated genetically and be made to produce therapeutically useful substances. This shows that bacteriology as a subject continues to thrive. It has many tentacles entwining with those of immunology, with clinical diagnosis and with antibiotic and chemical therapy. It has a settled background of established techniques, which are constantly expanding and are being modified.

The twentieth century successes of bacteriology have at least in part been misleading to the rest of medicine. This phase has now passed, but it can be imagined that intellectual over-reaction led to ideas that all diseases would have one single cause and that that cause would operate as an attack of some sort arising outside the body. This, in fact, is a very useful general concept, but seems not to be universally true. This could, of course, have been easily predicted as a false assumption, but it is the way of the medical profession and of scientists to over-react in the first instance to new discoveries. They are taken up enthusiastically both in their specific and in their general aspects and overplayed. A reaction then sets in as failures accrue and gradually the new discoveries fall into their more rightful place in the scheme of things.

Interestingly enough part of the downfall of this general vaguely held notion arose from the other component of microbiology—virology. The idea of infecting organisms smaller than the bacteria had arisen quite early in the twentieth century. The Rickettsiae are indeed smaller, but it seemed likely that there were smaller organisms still. In certain sexually transmitted diseases such as that of granuloma inquinale Charles Donovan (1863–1951) had shown the presence of what he called inclusion bodies in the cells of the lesions. This was one of the earlier demonstrations of an organism getting inside a cell and re-directing its activities away from the normal.

It is now known that a virus can insinuate itself into the genetic mechanisms and change them so that the cell has new functions imposed on it, or it may die. This is true in a wide variety of diseases such as poliomyelitis, measles, mumps, rubella, smallpox, warts and verrucae and a host of others. This understanding has led on to the notions of viruses causing certain cancers and congenital defects. Viruses consist of certain ribonucleic acids of similar kinds to those present in the genes of the chromosomes which are in every cell. In 1910 Simon Flexner (1863–1946) of America had transmitted poliomyelitis to monkeys by injecting into them a cell-free filtrate of the nervous system of people dying of the disease. There was thus some very small particle that caused the disease. For a long time viruses were always referred to as filtrable. The following year Francis Peyton Rous (1879–1970) found a malignant tumour in fowls called a sarcoma which was transmitted from bird to bird like an infection or by cell-free filtrates of tumours when injected experimentally. This was among the first pieces of evidence that tumours might be caused by an environmental agent. Before about that time it seemed that many tumours simply arose *de novo* owing to some unexplained metabolic or other process of the body itself. The Rous sarcoma, however, simply remained a curiosity for a long time. Now Denis Burkitt (Contemporary) has shown that a human nasopharyngeal tumour, found in Africa, is ultimately caused by a viral infection carried to sufferers by insect bites.

It seems that many other malignant tumours may be shown in future to be similarly caused by viruses, so thoughts about causes have shifted from considerations of purely internal changes to those introduced from outside. Again there may be an over-reaction in pursuing the practical outcomes of this belief, for even if the body cells are assaulted from without some form of response is required from them for a tumour to result. All disease is compounded of action and reaction. So all disease processes are multifactorial. There is no single cause for any single disease. This is a truism now but it has taken time to arrive at it and have it sink into the unconscious of the collective mind of medicine.

It is intriguing once again to note how bacteriology and virology intertwine with so many other fields of biological and medical endeavour. From the apparently simple idea of organisms attacking the body from outside there have grown the concepts and experiments of bodily responses which move into immunology, genetics and cancer. Despite all the specialization the boundaries between the specialties have to be crossed and re-crossed and concepts in one field are fecund in others and vice versa. At an even more general level it is worth a mention that viruses are relatively simple (in the biological sense) chemical substances. They can almost be kept in a jar like any other substance in a chemical laboratory. Yet when they are introduced into a living body they begin to take over some parts of it and replicate. The one essential feature of life is that of multiplication and reproduction. Here it would seem are chemical substances normally thought of as non-living, which in the right environment take on the characteristics of life. This is another indication that the boundary between the living and the non-living is not precise. The division is only broadly true, not totally so. It is a first reasonable assumption to be made by human minds, but no more. Like all such generalizations it needs much qualification in order to get nearer to the truth.

The study of the blood and its diseases—haematology—is another branch of pathology that has become a specialty during the twentieth century. Its story is inseparable from physiology, respiration, immunology, oncology and indeed every branch of medicine. Blood is virtually everywhere in the body and is the medium for carriage of chemicals to and from all tissues. It has roles in defence, both cellular and humoral. It seems to have involvement in everything, in one way or another. Moreover, it is easy to sample and analyse in the laboratory. Small amounts removed by venepuncture, which is perhaps the commonest form of 'biopsy', can have estimations performed on them which are then indicative, and can be transposed to the whole volume of blood. It is an intriguing mixture, and even in mediaeval times it was known as the paramount humour among the four then thought to be the basis of all pathology. Vincenzo Menghini had found iron in the blood as early as 1746, and in 1797 William Charles Wells (1757–1817) showed that the iron was in a complex substance (subsequently named haemoglobin). And of course there was interest in clotting because of its strangeness in the instant change from fluid to solid as soon as the vascular system is breached. There had been many investigations of this during the nineteenth century. Ernst Felix Hoppe-Seyler (1825–1895) showed haemoglobin to be a crystalline substance. Ernst Neumann (1834–1918) showed that red cells and white cells were produced in the bone marrow, and dozens of others had found and named the various cellular elements in circulating blood. Paul Ehrlich (1854–1915) about 1879 had established the basis of the differential count of the cells.

On these various bases haematology was built in the twentieth century. Red cells have been measured, haemoglobin estimated, the functions of white cells established (especially the role of the lymphocytes in immunological responses), blood gases analysed and the functions of proteins have more readily been understood, and also those of the bone marrow. Malignant diseases of the blood have been characterized. The discovery of the reticuloendothelial system by Karl Albert Aschoff (1866–1942) in 1924 takes the haematologist into the investigation of organs of the body such as lymph nodes, spleen and liver as well as bone marrow. The mechanisms of clotting have been and continue to be unravelled. In fact blood coagulation has become a specialty in its own right. One step in the direction of understanding came from Jay McLean (1890–1957), who discovered heparin in 1916. In some circumstances this prevents clotting. Blood transfusion too is now a specialty, dating from the discovery of inherited blood groups by Karl Landsteiner (1868–1943) in 1901. And the further blood groups were discovered later in the century, including the Rhesus factor by Philip Levine and Rufus Stetson (Contemporaries) in 1939.

Arising out of the great advances in chemistry and physics as well as physiology and biochemistry has come chemical pathology, or clinical chemistry. Because it is so specialized and so all-pervading and rapidly advancing it is not possible to document anything specifically of it here. Tissue fluids are the environment of all cells. The fluids take from, add to and exchange with the blood. There are also urine, cerebrospinal fluid, amniotic fluid and various effusions into body cavities. Solid tissues can be minced or otherwise treated to make them suitable for chemical analysis. Drugs, hormones and proteins can be assayed because of advances in technology. It seems that everything can be investigated chemically.

All living processes have a chemical base and when they do go awry the first change is probably chemical within one, few or several cells. It is only at a much later stage that these chemical changes are of such magnitude that they express themselves in structural or disease terms. Indeed, many diseases are diagnosed by the clinical chemist before there are any changes that could be made visible to the naked eye or under the microscope. This is why chemical pathology and biochemistry have taken on a dominant role in medicine and biology. Chemistry is at the foundations of all branches of biology, including medicine. If abnormal chemical processes can be identified before structural changes in cells occur then there is apparently a chance of diverting the processes once more back to normality, and overt disease may then be prevented or its course cut short. This may be a dream, but it seems on the way to coming true. It is a dream not normally much recounted. It remains in the background, ever-present yet unobserved. There is belief in the power of chemistry to explain fundamentals and to help us get closer to the truth, partly because chemical substances are measurable. Thus chemistry and chemical pathology are often believed to be more in the mainstream of the methods of the natural sciences than subjects such as biology, psychology and sociology.

The pathological subjects of histopathology (morbid anatomy), microbiology, haematology and clinical chemistry are sometimes grouped together as being the scientific basis of medicine, or the science of disease. They have expanded and have added to the accuracy of diagnosis and treatment mainly in the twentieth century. They will continue to burgeon, and from the main branches will come more and more sub-specialties. It is inevitable in the growth of science and the increasingly specialized concepts and techniques feeding that growth. Pathology especially emphasizes this specialization, though all departments of medicine display it. Only in the very broadest terms can pathologists from different disciplines communicate accurately with one another. People from the clinical disciplines too have similar problems. There are erudite and esoteric professionals in each specialty, and external amateurs who partly play the same game, but often have to be spectators whom the specialists instruct at (for the professionals) superficial level so that they may have some inkling of what is going on. This problem of communication is real and unlikely to be fully solved. Yet the amateurs (professionals in their own subjects) must remain in touch with the professionals. The essential problem is how much do the amateurs need to know to be able to do so.

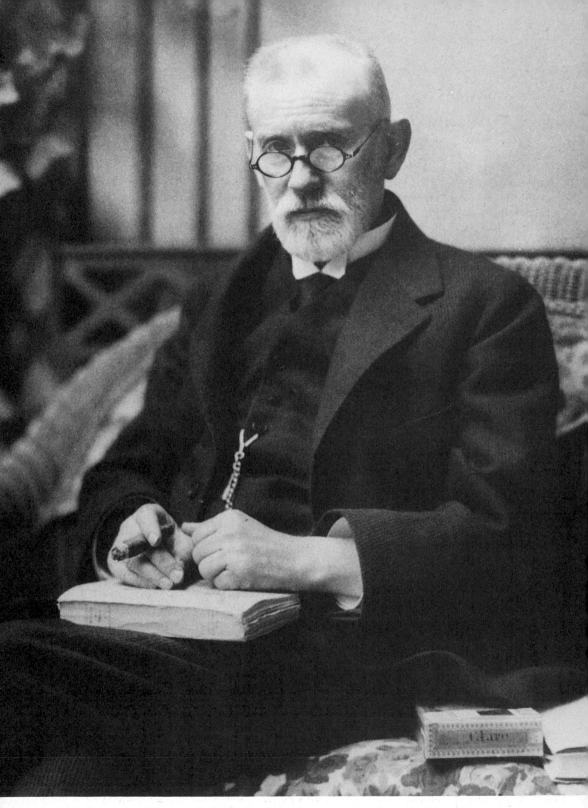

Paul Ehrlich, [1854–1915]. (Reproduced by courtesy of the Wellcome Institute Library, London)

138

Clinical Disciplines

The sub-heading of 'clinical disciplines' is in many senses misleading. It is intended to ease the task of the reader. To get a grip on concepts, knowledge has to be compartmentalized. In practice the departments of knowledge that we name are far from separate from each other. Knowledge is a nexus. It is so vast that we have to thread our way through it by selection of some items and groups of items so that we do not entirely lose our way. The apparently separate subjects are then landmarks from which we can get a bearing, but all landmarks can be seen from many different vantage points.

Many pathologists would class themselves as practising a specialty of clinical medicine. Pharmacologists too might well claim similarly. Physiology, anatomy, biochemistry, genetics, psychology, even physics and chemistry add to and take from clinical medicine. Classically this has meant bedside medicine in which a doctor deals with one patient at a time—a one-to-one relationship. This is now something of a rarity. Even when it appears to exist there is always a small or large team standing behind the doctor, waiting to be called into action should the patient's problems be deemed to need one, some or all of these additional helpers. The apparent simplicity of the older concept of what constitutes clinical medicine has largely dissolved in the inexorable growth of specialization. Yet for present purposes 'clinical disciplines' is a useful subdivision, for it implies a relationship of individual people with the medical process, rather than with physical parts of them in relative isolation. Even that is inexact, but the distinction will be enough for the present and will perhaps simplify consideration.

Medicine (physic), about the turn of the century, in both theory and practice, could be and was totally encompassed by individual physicians. Many clinical pictures were established as a basis for classification. The doctor was essentially a natural historian, watching the progress of diseases without much hope of altering their courses. The fact that doctors (and their patients) thought that medical interventions were valuable does not alter the present-day view. They were diagnosticians and prognosticians essentially, with a very weak therapeutic armamentarium which they did not recognize as such. There were opium and its derivatives, digitalis, purgatives of varying degrees of violence, herbs, metallic salts, expectorants of doubtful efficacy, linctuses, counter-irritants to rub on to the skin, stimulants and sedatives which were nearly all useless. The doctors practised in fact by using therapeutic folklore, based in botany and a largely valueless immense superstructure of materia medica and pharmacognosy, all of which have disappeared from the canon of medicine. They were left with counsel about diet, drink, bowel function, fresh air, cold, warmth and baths. They pontificated about healthy living and the avoidance of illness and its cure without much rational foundation for their beliefs. Only comparatively rarely could they bring about active harm by their advice. With careful watching and the passage of time the outcome could only be that of spontaneous cure, continuing disability or death.

Yet insight into clinical medicine was being heightened by the discoveries in bacteriology and in cellular pathology, both initiated mainly in the last quarter of the nineteenth century. Clinicians then and in the early decades of the twentieth century made their contributions to these subjects too. It was commonplace for them to be able to move from the bedside to the laboratory, where the clinician could master the relatively simple techniques as well as maintain his clinical expertise. Within his spheres he could be a jack-of-all-trades.

However, the splits into specialties were already beginning in the earlier decades of the twentieth century. Paul Ehrlich (1854–1915) with Sahachiro Hata (1873–1938) introduced the drug salvarsan, also called 606, because there had been this number of experiments to find a substance that would cure syphilis. Ehrlich was imbued with the idea that 'magic bullets' could be found for the cure of disease. They would be specific, and as regards acute infection the general concept has been found to be largely true. Before his time the treatment of syphilis was by mercury or bismuth, whereas salvarsan is a compound of arsenic. Similar such compounds have been found of value in some tropical diseases caused by protozoa, such as trypanosomiasis. The arsenical treatment of syphilis has been entirely superseded by newer antibiotics, but it held the field for about three decades. It was an important milestone in therapeutics for it showed that specific treatments could be found by tenacity of purpose and by much experimental trial and error.

With all the other advances taking place in the understanding and diagnosis of syphilis there came specialists in the venereal diseases. For a long time they practised dermatology as well, and in some parts of the world still do. The reason may be that several sexually transmitted diseases have cutaneous manifestations, and this can be especially marked in the secondary stage of syphilis. The disease was so rife until recently that the differential diagnosis of any skin rash had to include the possibility of syphilis. Venereology and dermatology were therefore among the earliest of specialties to begin to split off from general medicine. Now of course in most advanced countries even these two have separated from each other.

Another specialty of the twentieth century is cardiology. As a clinical discipline it has been built on such investigations as those of Wilhelm His jun. (1863–1934), who described the specialized conducting muscle of the heart in 1893; of Augustus Désiré Waller (1856–1922), who showed the electrical currents in the heart in 1887 which led to electrocardiography, now commonplace and much extended; of Pierre Carl Potain (1825–1901) of Paris, who measured the blood pressure routinely with a sphygmomanometer; of Sir James Mackenzie (1853–1925), who from 1892 in a series of researches analysed the pulse and cardiac rhythms in health and disease; of Lauder Brunton (1844–1916), who produced a textbook of pharmacology in 1885, in which amyl nitrite was described for its beneficial effects in angina pectoris. All of these are of interest in showing the way in which a medical specialty starts. There has to be an appropriate anatomical and physiological understanding together with a technology that makes diagnosis more precise and a therapy which can be seen to be of value. This last came with digitalis and amyl nitrite and the technology came with the sphygmomanometer, the polygraph for analysing the pulse and the electrocardiograph for analysing electrical activity in the heart. Later and further techniques have been added since the early days, as imaging and pressure recordings as well as clinical chemistry have become refined. And cardiac surgery, dating from about the mid-century, has acted on the medical advances and been acted on by them to make cardiology one of the most esoteric departments of medicine. The actions and reactions of clinical insight and understanding with technology are indivisible.

Respiratory diseases have become a specialty. Chest physicians had inherited the techniques of percussion from Auenbrugger and of auscultation from Laënnec in the nineteenth century as also had cardiology. Tuberculosis was especially rife early in the twentieth century and there were only natural cures to be hoped for. Patients were isolated in sanatoria, and put on a strict regimen, always including good food and fresh air. They needed doctors to look after them in these country places away from mainstream medicine, so that the physicians inevitably specialized. Then physiologists investigated respiratory function, in the lungs, in the blood and in the tissue cells and organs. A body of corporate knowledge became established and clinicians began to use the techniques and researches introduced by physiologists into spirometry, into gases in the lungs and blood and tissues, and into the nervous control of respiration. Various imaging techniques—based first in radiology and later allied with the ability to look down the bronchi and into the pleural cavity round the lungs—along with improving microbiology and histopathology extended the range of diagnosis, which has become more precise. Adding to this has been the extension of surgery safely into the thorax. This began about 1933 when Evarts Ambrose Graham (1883–1957) and Jacob Jesse Singer (1882–1954) in the USA described the first successful removal of a whole lung for carcinoma. It was not, however, until after the 1939–45 war that chest surgery became more commonplace because of advances in antibiotic therapy, blood transfusion and anaesthesia. The great variety of pulmonary infections came to light with the improvement and increase of microbiological techniques. Antibiotics helped differentiate these infections since some diseases were cured by them and not others, the latter therefore being highlighted as worthy of further investigation.

Like all other specialties chest medicine draws on a variety of concepts and techniques derived from other disciplines and turns them to its own ends. The total corpus of knowledge is such that only specialists can now cope with it and practise at a high level of expertise.

By 1900 neurological medicine had many useful descriptions of diseases and syndromes, showing some localization of function in the brain and spinal cord and so allowing of some fairly accurate diagnoses. It is a slight surprise to find, however, that Joseph François Félix Babinski (1857–1922) only described his reflex as late as 1896, and it is now an integral part of every clinical neurological examination of a patient. The basic sciences have helped enormously too. Over the years anatomists, especially with the help of electron microscopy, have delineated more and more tracts and nuclei. Physiologists and chemists have shown many of the characteristics of the nerve impulse both in the central and peripheral nervous systems, and how it has physical, electrical and chemical components. This has led to greatly increased understanding. Drugs have been introduced to help with some neuromuscular diseases. Pathological knowledge has assisted too in post-mortem and biopsy diagnosis. Radiological examination of the skull was written about by Artur Schüller (1874–1958) in 1912. Since then great strides have been made in imaging techniques by injections of contrast media into central nervous system spaces and lately by computerized axial tomography as well as by injections which show up the vascular tree on X-ray. Of course there has been continuing use of lumbar puncture, which was written about by Hans Heinrich Georg Queckenstedt (1876–1918) in 1916.

The precision of diagnosis has much increased, and great emphasis is now laid on rehabilitation when disease has impaired the patient's abilities. Although progress seems slow there have been some advances in therapy which have improved well-being and recovery in nervous system disease. These same advances have made their contribution to psychology and psychiatry. As the brain is the organ of the mind there has always been overlap in content between these various branches of science and medicine, and Jean-Martin Charcot (1825–1893) in Paris and Silas Weir Mitchell (1829–1914) in the USA are widely known for their work both in the physical and in the mental characteristics of brain disorder. The two aspects have largely separated during the twentieth century.

Neurosurgery has become a reality in this century. It is based in its own techniques of access to sites of pathology and those required to deal with lesions, whatever their nature. They can be called into play because of more precise diagnosis and localization of the seats of disease, and they have extended into the areas of the pituitary and therefore endocrine surgery and of surgery of the back, and there has been some taking over of the techniques of vascular surgery and of microsurgery to deal with intracranial and intraspinal lesions. The possibility of invasion of these delicate areas has come about because of advances, as before noted, in antibiotic therapy, blood transfusion and anaesthesia and knowledge of the pathophysiology of the recovery period after operation. In the sphere of neurosurgery it is impossible to leave out the name of Harvey Cushing (1869–1939), the doyen of the modern subject.

In a short history it is not sensible to try to document all the other specialties which have arisen in the twentieth century. Each has its own lengthy history to record. The patterns of development have all been similar in essence. First have come clinical and classic descriptions of disease and their classification. Then there has been a search for deeper understanding which may have come from anatomy, physiology, chemistry, physics, biochemistry and improved diagnostic technology, by imaging techniques and by clinical chemistry. There have come improved techniques also in visualizing body tubes and cavities directly through fibre-optic instruments. And there are recording instruments of great complexity based in electronics. There seems to be no end to the ingenuity displayed and brought to fruition, so that ultimately all may use routinely what were once only research tools. Moreover the process is world-wide, with rapid diffusion of what is learned by communication and the information industries.

The success story of the twentieth century has been the near conquest of infections of many kinds. At the opening of the century infections were among the major killing diseases, especially of the young. Prevention was in its infancy through sanitary engineering and public health control of water and food supplies, and isolation of patients was practised to try to control the spread of infection. Yet there was no specific remedy with which to combat infections once contracted. Reliance had to be placed on non-specific measures and natural resistance. Then came salvarsan for syphilis in 1906. Nothing further of worth happened until 1936 when Gerhard Domagk (1895–1964) introduced Prontosil Rubrum, which was the first of the sulphonamides. For this he was awarded the Nobel Prize in 1939. This drug transformed the prognosis in a wide variety of bacterial diseases, including those caused by pneumococci, streptococci and staphylococci. These often had a very high mortality, but now the majority became curable and cured. The pharmaceutical companies went to work to manufacture and market new drugs in the same series of sulphonamides. Many of them came to practical use. The companies were able to do this because of the advances that had been made in physics, chemistry and chemical engineering. The drugs had a part to play in the prosecution of the war of 1939–45. Troops were rapidly cured of dysentery, that decimator of armies, and so could return to the battlefronts with minimum delay. When they were injured they could be brought more safely to surgery and so might be cured or at least spared, with less maiming than they otherwise might have had. The new drugs were scarcely believable in their impact and efficacy. They wrought a change in thinking about the way in which disease might be cured and conquered. A previously impossible dream became reality.

Despite their value the sulphonamides were soon found to have some drawbacks, especially in unpleasant side-effects on the blood and kidneys. Then came penicillin, which by comparison was virtually harmless. Alexander Fleming (1881–1955) (*Figure 10.3*) in 1929 had found that some of his laboratory cultures of bacteria had been inhibited in their growth by a mould called penicillium. Such contamination and its effects had been noted by others on many occasions, but there was then no attempt made to turn this observation into therapeutic effect. This was done by Ernst Boris Chain (1906–1979) and Howard Florey (1898–1968) working in Oxford, England (*Figure 10.4*). Their work was published in 1940, and no doubt was pressed forward by the needs of war and of traumatic surgery. All three were awarded the Nobel Prize in 1945. Again the work was seminal and prompted a search by pharmaceutical companies and others for similar valuable substances. Now the chemical structure of penicillin is known, and the molecule has

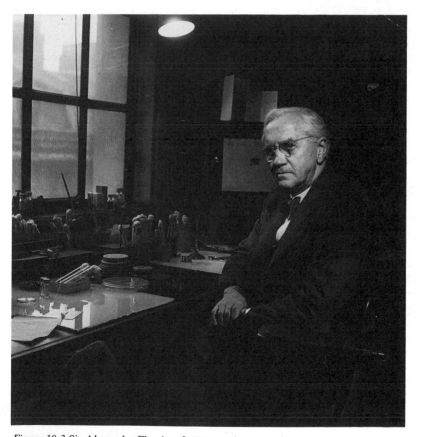

Figure 10.3 Sir Alexander Fleming. [1881–1955]. (Reproduced by courtesy of the BBC Hulton Picture Library, London)

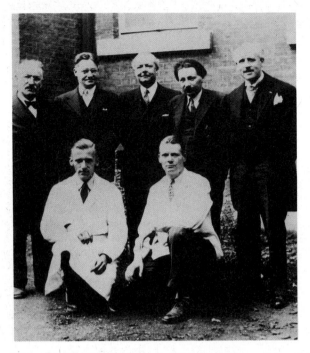

Figure 10.4 Antibiotics pioneers at Oxford. Back row, L top: S. Waksman, H. Florey, J. Trefouel, E. B. Chain, A. Gratia. Front row: P. Fredericq and Maurice Welsch. (Reproduced by courtesy of the Wellcome Institute Library, London)

been manipulated in many ways which have produced a range of penicillins of therapeutic value. And more and more antibiotics have been found since, with streptomycin in 1944, chloramphenicol in 1947, aureomycin in 1948, cephalosporin in 1948 and many others later.

The dependence of these discoveries on other disciplines requires no further emphasis. Many of them were pressed into service and they are still being raided for the contributions to medicine that they might bring. The finding and testing of these antibiotics requires great resources of energy, enthusiasm, facilities, but above all money. Only advanced countries with a healthy economy can carry out such searches and testing. This explains some of the importance of wealthy pharmaceutical companies which have flourished since the war of 1939–45.

To have virtually controlled infection, where money is available to pay for medicine at an advanced level, is an immense achievement, made over only about 40 years. It cannot be said that all infections are controlled, but the vast majority are. Some virus infections, in particular, are not yet susceptible to treatment by antibiotics, but many are preventable. A major approach to this has been by the use of vaccines, in the tradition of Edward Jenner. His vaccinations against smallpox were built on an empirical foundation. Now with better understanding of immune responses it is possible to be more rational in research into making vaccines. The general system of attempting to cure by vaccines had been extended into bacterial diseases in the early years of the twentieth century, and prominent among those using this method was Almroth Wright at St. Mary's Hospital, London, where Fleming was one of his pupils. The coming of the range of antibiotics for the treatment of bacterial infections has tended to make vaccine treatment for them increasingly superfluous. But for viral infections therapeutic agents have not been so successful. They will be, however. Already there are a few showing promise (interferon, acyclovir) and such is the power of physics, chemistry, biology and technology that it can only be a matter of time before viral infections come under control by specific therapy.

Among the more important vaccines for prevention of infection are those for poliomyelitis and rubella. Jonas Edward Salk (1914–) in 1953 introduced a vaccine for infantile paralysis, and as a result the ravages of this disease have been much reduced world-wide. His work arose out of knowing the natural history of polio, together with the improvement in the laboratory techniques of virology, such that poliovirus could be grown and attenuated under laboratory conditions. The disease is now preventable, though mass vaccination of susceptible populations is not everywhere politically and economically possible. This interface between valid research findings and putting them to practical effect is still one of difficulty; it is that of social action being pressed forward for the sake of the individual members of society. However, this has been effective for smallpox, for in the 1970s the disease was eradicated, probably never to return. This came about because the spread of the virus is from person to person without any intermediate vector and because all countries of the world initiated and maintained vaccination programmes helped by the World Health Organization, which was set up in 1948. The spread of the virus was therefore blocked everywhere by vaccinated populations and so the virus has been unable to survive. Its environment was made so inimical that it had nowhere to go and nothing it could exploit.

Norman McAlister Gregg (1892–1966), an opthalmologist of Australia, in 1940 found a cluster of children with congenital cataract. Following this up he found that their mothers had contracted German measles (rubella) in pregnancy. It emerged that this disease could affect the embryo so that the resultant children might have congenital defects in the eyes, ears and heart. The finding was staggering for it showed that congenital abnormality could be caused by environmental factors. Before then it had been believed that all such abnormalities were due to some inherent defect in the genetic mechanisms. The whole attitude to genetic abnormalities changed in a very short time. Apart from anything else there was the possibility of prevention, which prior to this time had been thought impossible. Prevention, in fact, came very quickly, for a vaccine against rubella was produced; and it became possible to diagnose the illness accurately by serological methods. Mass vaccination programmes directed at young girls and pregnant women and those likely to become pregnant have vastly reduced the load of congenital disease caused by rubella. Similar attempts have been made to produce vaccines to prevent other virus diseases such as measles and mumps, but not so far with the success attending vaccination against rubella, smallpox and polio. Against bacteria, however, there are successes in the prevention of tetanus, typhoid and whooping cough, and many others.

The majority of bacterial diseases are now curable by antibiotics or other chemotherapeutic agents when illness strikes the individual. Many virus diseases, formerly killers, are preventable by vaccination, and curative agents are probably on the way fairly soon. The more non-specific measures of public health and hygiene, with improved living conditions, must not be forgotten. They began to have their effects in reducing mortality before the specific drugs were available. The attack on infections has to be many pronged, so that the dramatic effects of antibiotics must not be allowed completely to overshadow the more humdrum approaches. They are more obviously in evidence in some tropical diseases, where an understanding of the natural history has led to campaigns designed to kill insect vectors such as mosquitoes and flies, which convey malaria, filaria, yellow fever, gastrointestinal and other diseases. In bilharziasis an intermediate host is the snail. All these carriers of disease can be attacked and kept under control by drainage of their breeding grounds, by proper disposal of human and other excreta and by destroying vectors by chemical means, of which the outstanding example is DDT, introduced in large measure by Paul Müller (1899–1965) about 1944. For this he received the Nobel Prize in 1948. And of course there have been advances in the treatment, as distinct from prevention, of many of the protozoal diseases and other infecting agents especially inhabiting the tropics and subtropics.

The rapidity of air travel has led to several small outbreaks of such diseases in temperate climates, when sufferers or vectors have been introduced there unwittingly. Various national and international controls have therefore been introduced to prevent the spread of infections. The price of control of infection is eternal vigilance both in prevention and in cure. All available methods of control have to be used.

There is a tendency to concentrate attention almost exclusively on individual patients in hospital beds, and it must be resisted in the interests of real understanding of how infectious disease must always be combated on a variety of fronts. A large book could be written on this subject alone, but this brief outline must suffice here. And there is the message that the classic physician at the bedside is by no means the only person to be involved, so that where a 'clinical' or 'non-clinical' subject now ends is not clear cut.

The antibiotics for the treatment of infections are part of the study of pharmacology, which has made enormous strides in the twentieth century. Hormones have been mentioned in connection with physiology, but they have also been introduced into medical treatment with great success. Insulin for the treatment of diabetes has been referred to, and also thyroid preparations for myxoedema (thyroid deficiency). The discovery of hormones of the steroid series in the adrenal glands has led to quite new approaches to the management of certain joint diseases, especially rheumatoid arthritis. It was the amelioration of this disease in pregnancy that caused Edward Calvin Kendall (1886–1972) and his colleagues to search for the hormone bringing about this effect. In 1934 they found cortin. This was followed very rapidly by the discovery of several steroid compounds, not only of value in arthritis but also essential for life support, the control of mineral and of carbohydrate metabolism, and the control of many sexual and reproductive functions. The steroid compounds are built into the very stuff of cellular physiology and pathology, and they have been found in the lowliest of plant and animal species and throughout the animal kingdom. Study of them is more than a lifetime's work. They are now in use medically every day for substitution therapy when the natural secretions are deficient, and there are also antagonists to various steroid and other hormones when these are secreted excessively and become the causes of disease.

Hormones have been extracted both from anterior and from posterior parts of the pituitary gland and have found use in labour, in control of water excretion, in stimulating growth when it is deficient, and in the higher control of the thyroid and adrenal glands. Part of the integration of the endocrine system resides in the pituitary hormones, so that their effects in therapy are widespread and often helpful. Further research has shown how the hypothalamus controls pituitary function, and hormones have been characterized from this part of the brain so that they can be used therapeutically. And more than this it is possible to produce antibodies to some of these powerful molecules so that any excess production of them may be diminished or even eliminated. Similar advances have been made in the understanding and therapeutic control of the parathyroid glands, concerned with calcium and phosphate levels in the blood and therefore of importance in the maintenance of the skeleton, of proper excitability in nerve and muscle, and in kidney function.

In the ovaries and testes steroid hormones are part of the essence of maleness and femaleness. Combined contraceptive pills, combined because they consist of two types of hormone, are in use by millions of women throughout the world. The effect was demonstrated first by Gregory Goodwin Pincus (1903–1967) in 1953. It opened up an entirely new field in birth control and prevention, which still has not been fully explored. Its social repercussions and the changes it has helped to bring about in sexual mores are still with us and many of the problems it has brought in its train have not been resolved. The understanding and the technology have been magnificent, but they have posed serious questions outside the immediate field of medicine.

The pharmacological revolution has extended beyond all previously conceived bounds. The pharmacopoeia of 1940 bears little resemblance to that of 1980. Advances in physics, chemistry, biochemistry, physiology, immunochemistry and a host of other disciplines have made this possible. When chains of metabolic processes begin to be understood it can often be conjectured where they might be going wrong and to make guesses as to how they might be put right. Then it is possible to make new compounds to insert into metabolic processes, such that there is a likelihood of influencing them. This comes about partly because of an understanding of the importance of molecular shapes and how various parts of the jigsaws fit into one another. Pharmacology therefore becomes rationally directed rather than a matter of trial and error, which Ehrlich had to practise with salvarsan. Many new drug discoveries are marvels of the use of knowledge and technology to reach desired and directed ends. In no previous century was this possible and it has arisen out of concepts and technology and their developments dating from the end of the nineteenth century and into the present one.

The story of molecular structure and its importance in biological function and process is particularly exemplified by enzymes. These are the ubiquitous substances, mainly of protein type, that direct cellular metabolic processes by locking on to other molecules because of their shapes, as a spanner fits on to a nut or the head of a bolt, or as a key into a lock. The molecules are then made to break up or be re-arranged or be latched on to others.

Enzymes are like workers on an assembly line, putting together and taking apart in continuous process, yet they only facilitate that process and are not incorporated directly into it. Like the workers they tend to stay in the same station, make one adjustment to the assembly and then the partly finished product is moved to the next point. Understanding began with Claude Bernard in the nineteenth century, and in 1897 Eduard Buchner (1860–1907) showed that fermentation was possible without the presence of whole cells, such as those of yeast. In other words fermentation (a metabolic process) must basically be chemical. Then in 1909 Archibald Edward Garrod (1857–1936) wrote his *Inborn Errors of Metabolism*, which went into a second edition in 1923, and was reprinted in 1963. This described a series of congenital biochemical abnormalities (such as alkaptonuria and cystinuria) in which the cause was essentially the absence of an enzyme so that a particular metabolic process was blocked. The result could be an overt disease. This is well shown by phenylketonuria, described in 1934 by Ivor Følling (1888–1973). In this the metabolism of a protein is blocked by the absence of an enzyme, phenylalanine hydroxylase. Phenylalanine and other products accumulate in the blood, and children who have the disease may suffer from mental retardation. Now several thousand enzymes are known, and it is certain that each of us is deficient in some, but fortunately it seems to be only a few that cause disease when lacking.

This all begins to tie in with genetics, and with the whole of cellular biology. The genes on the chromosomes which are in the nucleus of every cell are made up of DNA in the form of a double helix. The arrangement of the four nucleic acids along this double chain determines which proteins, including enzymes, shall be manufactured. The 'message' is taken on by messenger RNA (ribonucleic acid) which functions in the cytoplasm of the cell outside the nucleus. In the cytoplasm is an astonishing factory, for it is made up of a complex series of assembly lines on sinuous membranes, with little knots of activity, called ribosomes, strung out along them. And there is a sort of powerhouse in the mitochondria of each cell. All these are the subcellular organelles, whose structure has been elucidated mainly with the use of the electron microscope.

The chains of many metabolic processes are now worked out. Among the earlier ones were those for carbohydrate metabolism, of protein and fat cycles, and now they are characterized for many secretions and hormones. It is an astonishing edifice to have built in so short a time. There can be no wonder that specialization has become necessary, in the face of such exponentially expanding knowledge and technology. Even more than in preceding centuries it is obvious that dozens, perhaps hundreds, of scientists and doctors are pursuing roughly similar courses in their thoughts and investigations, so that sometimes there comes a race to be the first to publish a new discovery. But whatever is published is not the work of one person. It rests on an enormously large supporting team, scattered throughout many laboratories, universities, research institutes and hospitals. Each member of the team may give a touch to the ball to allow one person to score the goal, and the scorer may not even know or be aware of those who have made his success possible. There is a public unperceived intellectual environment surrounding all who work in a particular discipline. They draw on it and add to it without always being aware that they do. Nothing happens in isolation from this environment.

It should not be necessary to re-emphasize that these researches have had a profound effect on clinical medicine. They have helped to disentangle groups of diseases only previously delineated clinically. Every clinical disease category has expanded into more and more subcategories as understanding at ever deeper levels of chemistry, immunology, genetics and other disciplines has increased. Important nuances of disease processes come to light at these deeper levels and they cannot be inferred from consideration of the natural history of disease as observed by the physician. His tasks have been eased in one direction by deeper understanding and by the help of colleagues in the laboratories and diagnostic clinics. At the same time the task has become more difficult because of the vast amount of information he receives both in general and about his individual patients. Not only is this true for the 'basic' sciences, for he must also take account of the psychology of his patients and of the sociological components of their disorders, as will emerge subsequently.

All this information has to be reduced to some sort of order and put in some scale of importance for each patient to be helped to solve his problems. The twentieth century has brilliantly succeeded in many aspects of clinical medicine, but these have drawn attention to yet more and more questions to be answered. Complexity becomes compounded.

Diagnosis has become more precise and more time consuming. Imaging techniques have been mentioned. Direct viewing of the interiors of the body by clever optical methods have also. There are physical methods too in electroencephalography (brain waves), in tonometry of the eye (to measure the pressure within), in audiometry (to test hearing precisely), in electrocardiography (to display the currents generated by the heart), in cardiac catheterization (to measure pressure in the heart and great blood vessels), in respirometry (to measure pressures and flows of air in the lungs and their passages), in instruments to measure pressures in all parts of the alimentary tract, in similar ones for the urinary system, and also for the genital system, especially the uterus in labour. It is worth noting that sometimes these various instruments have refined simple clinical insight derived from observation. They have allowed interpretation of symptoms and signs with greater precision by the clinician, so that the instruments may no longer be needed.

On the other hand, the technologies may breed like rabbits as attempts are made to improve them and extract more and more information about what is happening to the patient. This leads to difficulties in transposing what is recorded to the understanding of the patient. What is the machine exactly telling the doctor? Is the machine in fact introducing sources of error? Only continued experiment can begin to answer these fundamental questions. Until there are closer approaches to the truth some patients will inevitably suffer because of ignorance of the doctors as to what it is that they are observing and interpreting. But this is no different from what it has always been. Medicine is always experiment. Hippocrates was experimenting with every patient he dealt with. There is no absolutely certain corpus of medicine that any instructed person can apply. Patients with similar diseases are not all the same. They will therefore not always respond in the same way to treatment. Even the simplest drug administered to several patients will not always bring about the same response in each. This ought to be apparent from the earlier considerations of genetics and of enzymes and proteins. No individual is exactly like any other in his basic metabolism. Whatever is done to him is therefore always an experiment. The outcome may, on the basis of previous experience and statistical evidence, be the usual one, but there is no certainty that a particular patient will conform with the average.

This completely unique individuality is too frequently ignored or forgotten by doctors and by those who criticize the directions in which they believe medicine is heading. Every intervention is an experiment because the full nature of the patient is never completely known or understood, even with all our present knowledge, nor is it ever likely to be. Medicine is an indeterminate art, however much scientists and the public would prefer it not to be. Whatever the consensus may be about the core of medicine in diagnosis and treatment, there will always be uncertainty at the heart of it because of personal uniqueness.

Medicine has become powerful in what it can do in diagnosis and in treatment, but as in everything else, such power is not an unmitigated boon, though that is what it would appear to be at first sight. Because patients differ from one another some medicines produce undesirable side-effects, so causing illness, disability and death. It is thought that up to about 20 per cent of patients admitted to hospital may be suffering from iatrogenic (doctor-caused) disorders. And with real power to influence events, such as only the twentieth century has given, there comes the problems of whether to use the power in every case and of when to stop intervention, because of humane reasons. The now classic example is that of patients with brainstem death who have no chance of real life and living, but whose hearts, lungs and kidneys can be made to function by a variety of techniques, drawing on many background sciences and technology. There is then the semblance of life in heartbeat, respiration, excretion and other body functions, but on any sensible definition the patient is dead.

The question becomes one of when or even whether to switch off the life-support systems. It is at points like these that thoroughgoing, purely scientific medicine has no answers within its own canon. The questions have moved into a quite different sphere of human thought and culture, and it is then that people outside medicine quite rightly feel that they must enter the lists and have an opinion and a voice. The nature of the problem will be explored further in a later chapter of this book.

To the unsophisticated it is surgery that has made the most spectacular advances in recent decades. The reason is probably that it has a mystique and a ritual which has some chance of being understood. The principles of surgery are relatively simple and straightforward. The disorders with which it deals are usually fairly localized. The offending lesion can then be removed. To do this there has to be a planned access, and a phase of ablation followed by one of repair. In their essence surgical tools are such that any carpenter and seamstress could comprehend. This does not belittle master craftsmen for there is much difference between an understanding within narrow limits and the actual carrying out of a surgical operation (or the making of a piece of furniture or dress). The conceptualizing of medicine (physic) and its therapeutic methods is more difficult than that of surgery for the amateur. The focus of thinking about surgery is the operating theatre, where in imagination the drama of life and death is played out. This ignores the bases on which surgery now rests. It is these that have made surgical intervention possible in more and more parts of the body. Only recently has it become reasonably safe to invade the chest to operate on lungs, heart, great vessels and oesophagus, and to invade the head and spinal column to deal with lesions of the nervous system. These invasions have been made possible by progress in anaesthesia, in blood transfusion and in the control of infection.

Haemorrhage and infection, as well as pain, have always been the most daunting problems for the surgeon and his patients. Anaesthesia was the first subject to advance to make surgery more bearable. The first steps were taken in the last half of the nineteenth century, in America and in Scotland, and also London. The improvements in the twentieth century have been in the finding of more and more anaesthetic agents, and much of this has been due to the activities of pharmaceutical companies, basing their work on pharmacological principles and chemistry, some of which have been enunciated earlier. The chemical characterization of known anaesthetics and analgesics have shown what sorts of molecules to look for and manufacture. Nitrous oxide, oxygen and ether were administered at operations through various forms of dispenser like that of Joseph Thomas Clover (1825–1882) in 1876. Towards the end of the 1914–18 war Henry Edmund Gaskin Boyle (1875–1941) produced a much better anaesthetic machine, which in principle has held the field since. It needed physics, chemistry, engineering technology, physiology, anatomy and biochemistry to make it valuable. The delivery of gases directly into the trachea, by passing a tube through the vocal cords, has made delivery to the right place more certain; and by having an inflatable cuff surrounding the tube, controlled positive-pressure anaesthesia became possible and at the same time prevented vomit gaining access to the lungs, an accident that can be disastrous. The technical aspects of delivery of anaesthetic gases have therefore overcome many of the problems earlier encountered.

New gases such as trichlorethylene, divinyl ether, cyclopropane and halothane have been introduced, as well as many others. Of equal importance has been the use of muscle relaxants, which have increased the range of surgery. Much of the difficulty of surgical access is due to muscle contractions inseparable from light anaesthesia. D-tubocurarine chloride was isolated from curare (used as a poison on arrow tips by South American Indians) in 1935 by Harold King (1887–1956). It was introduced into anaesthetic practice in 1942. Seven years later Daniel Bovet (1907–) brought in succinyl choline as a relaxant. Further help to the surgeon was given by the introduction of intravenous anaesthetics, the most valuable for its time being the barbiturate, thiopentone sodium or pentothal—reported on by John Silas Lundy (1894–) of the USA in 1935. This, and similar substances, allied with gases and relaxants have transformed surgery.

Proceeding at the same time were researches into the blocking of painful nerve impulses conveyed along peripheral nerves and also in the central nervous system. The first of such substances was cocaine (also used by South American Indians). This can be used as a spray on mucous membranes such as those of the nose and mouth, but when injected round nerves or into the spinal canal it can bring about anaesthesia; but it has its dangers. Other less dangerous substances have now been found such as procaine. Virtually any part of the body can now be anaesthetized by these locally acting chemicals, without any need for the patient to be unconscious, which is the necessary state when gases are used, for they act on the higher centres of the nervous system. The majority of patients and surgeons, however, prefer general anaesthesia, not wishing for a person to be conscious while his or her body is being operated on. Nevertheless, conduction anaesthesia has a place in many smaller operations or where there may be danger associated with affecting respiration, the heart or central nervous system, as general anaesthetics do.

The great range of anaesthetic agents and techniques means that operations lasting several hours can be undertaken. These are necessary in many such as those on the heart, lungs, nervous system, in trauma and in transplantation. Not only does the anaesthetist then require his direct anaesthetic skills, he has to call on those derived from metabolism and the physiology and pathology of all vital organs to keep his patient safe. It is therefore not surprising that his field has extended into pre- and postoperative care, thus trying to make the patient safe for surgery and its immediate aftermath. In this he is one of a team which includes the surgeon. As a result there has come increasing specialization in anaesthesia, for the problems of operations on different systems of the body have their own intricacies. The technology of the operating theatre which surrounds and is directed by the anaesthetist has demanded the training of special non-medical technicians to deal with it, especially when it goes wrong, as all machinery at some time will. When the technology was simple it was the province of the doctor and an anaesthetic nurse to maintain it. This is no longer possible. The nurse is still present but her task is to see to the general welfare and comfort of the patient. The technician copes with the technology, while the doctor has the general overview of his province.

Because many of the immediate problems and complications after surgical operation occur in the heart and lungs the anaesthetist has tended to be the one

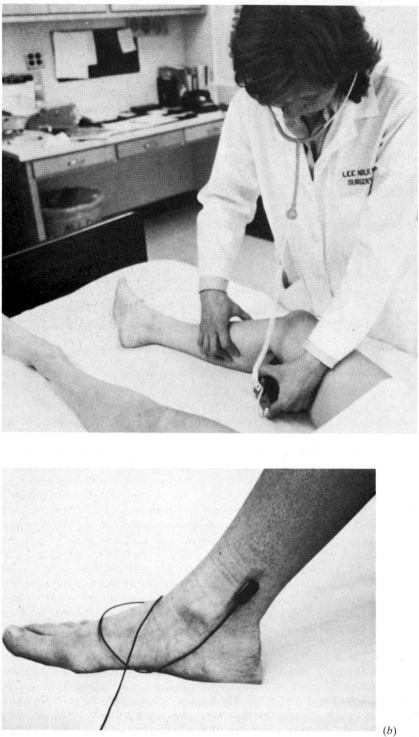

(a)

(b)

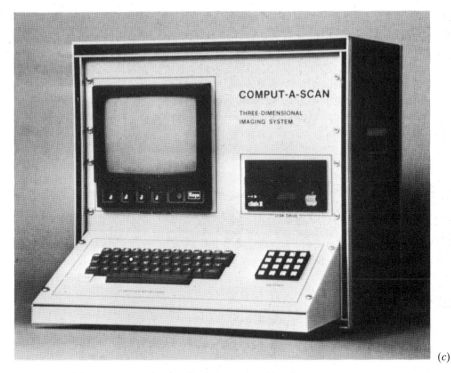

(c)

Figure 10.5 (a) Doppler examination for deep venous thrombosis.
(b) Use of polyplethysmograph for measurement of blood flow.
(c) Instrument that interfaces with a Hokanson pulsed-Doppler arteriograph for the production of multiplanar images. (From *Noninvasive Diagnosis of Vascular Disease*, 1984, reproduced by courtesy of Appleton Davies)

mainly in charge of the intensive care units, which have sprung up as adjuncts to the operating theatres. In these the immediate postoperative care is practised until the patient is fit enough to be returned to more general care. In the units again there has been specialization so that doctors, nurses and technicians are all needed, supported by the laboratory teams and diagnostic services. All this is a far cry from the 'rag and bottle' days of anaesthesia. This is exactly what it was. An ill-fitting mask of gauze was placed over the nose and mouth of the patient, and then the anaesthetic agent, choloroform or ether, was dripped on to the mask and the patient went to sleep. It is the anaesthetic progression that has been one of the major factors in making modern surgery possible, and with increasing safety for the patient. The surgeon has an inert patient on whose body he can operate. His concern at this time is purely corporeal and material. He is now given the chance to exercise his skill in a way never before possible.

The dramatic interlude of the actual operation in the surgical care of the patient is now not enough. Much work has to be done in the preoperative period to 'make the patient safe for surgery', and also in the postoperative period to deal with the problems arising out of the surgical intervention, and any continuing disease that there might be. This postoperative period has acute phases (following in the first few days after operation) and more chronic phases when the patient is convalescing both in the protected environment of the hospital and afterwards at home, or in the workplace. The surveillance is therefore intense at first and gradually becomes less as time passes. In both pre- and postoperative phases the psychological components of the patient's suffering have become increasingly recognized. This has only been possible because the physical problems of operation have been largely overcome.

The groups where psychological support is most necessary were early identified as those undergoing amputations of limbs, mastectomy in women, transplants, and plastic surgery around the head, neck and face. But these have led to greater recognition of the fact that all patients undergoing surgery of any type have psychological reactions to their diseases, their disabilities and operation which may be very disturbing to them. The disturbance can be minimized by explanations, assurance, kindly attitudes, understanding and patience on the part of helpers. This is simple preventive psychotherapy, which is interesting to see imported into what heretofore was thought of purely as a craft. Craftsmanship alone is not enough when dealing with people rather than physical materials.

The application of nutritional knowledge, previously referred to, has also helped in the better preparation of patients for surgery. Malnutrition may so debilitate as to make it difficult for the patient to withstand a surgical onslaught, may make him prone to infection afterwards and to failure of his wounds to heal. Much attention is therefore given to improving each patient's nutrition, when warranted, before operation, so that he shall be in the best possible condition for the particular surgery envisaged. This has undoubtedly helped to improve results, especially in major operations, and in very prolonged ones. Among the most important aspects of nutrition have been those of water, salt and other mineral metabolism. Owen Harding Wangensteen (1898–1981) in 1932 decompressed obstructed bowel by suction and this began the clinical investigations into losses of salts and water, so that now (1984) the correction of their balances by chemical analysis followed by appropriate infusions is routine. All these processes of control of nutrition also extend into convalescence.

There is concern too with respiration, cardiac function, excretion and other processes, both before and after operation. Although the surgical attack is concentrated on a relatively localized part of the body, the results may be diffused throughout the whole person in his mental and bodily functions. The concern with the whole person has always been characteristic of the best surgeons. Now the concern is being built into the practice of an increasing number of them, and this must be counted as an advance rivalling those in surgical techniques.

The control of bleeding has been the concern of surgeons over the centuries. It was classically done by pressure of fingers, pads and bandages and tourniquets, as well as by ligature of vessels and suturing. In essence they remain. Spencer Wells (1818–1897) introduced his forceps in 1879, and they greatly simplified the temporary control of bleeding until the vessels they held in their teeth could be ligatured or cauterized. All this is only necessary because the clots that finally seal the vessels take time to form. Naturally there have been experiments to attempt to make such clotting occur more rapidly, in the final hope that surgeons might cut blood vessels with comparative impunity and not have their view of the operative field obscured by blood. But the problem is tricky in that what is needed is clotting when the vessel is severed but not while the blood is circulating. Blood clots (thrombosis) within main arteries and veins are serious and may be lethal. Instruments that coagulate the blood as the vessels are cut have included diathermy (high-frequency electric current) and laser beams. They have their drawbacks, but no doubt others will be introduced. But the really major advances have been in correcting anaemia in patients prior to operation, and in replacing blood lost by injury, disease or operation by transfusion. The intention is to maintain the total blood volume of the patient within relatively narrow limits.

Transfusion was attempted in earlier centuries between animals and between humans and animals. They had to be direct from the vessels of the donor to those of the recipient. They were not generally successful. The change began when blood was withdrawn into a vessel from the donor and then poured into the recipient using rubber tubing and a funnel. And the invention of the hollow needle must not be forgotten as a necessity now in transfusion and a variety of other procedures. The reasons for failure of earlier attempts became clearer with Landsteiner's description of blood groups in 1901 and of Landsteiner and Wiener's discovery of the Rhesus factor in 1940. After many vicissitudes over the intervening years transfusions are given that are compatible as between donors and recipients, and they are safe. It became possible to store blood when prevention of coagulation on collection was brought in by adding sodium citrate and glucose, a method used by Albert Hustin (1882–1967) and reported in 1914. The war gave an enormous fillip to transfusion, and citrated blood was widely used for the injured. It was in 1917–18 that Oswald Hope Robertson (1886–1966) used it after storing for casualties on the battlefield. The first blood bank in peacetime was established at Cook County Hospital, Chicago, in 1937 by Bernard Fantus (1874–1940). Now of course there are blood banks everywhere, and in the UK organized by the National Blood Transfusion Service. This came firmly into being during the war of 1939–45.

Blood transfusion is now a specialty and it has widened in scope because blood obtained from donors is used as a source of myriad therapeutic agents. It is an immensely complex fluid, and modern techniques have allowed the extraction and purification of a whole host of substances of value in treatment.

The final base from which surgery has taken off is that of the control of infection. This began with Lister and antisepsis and then moved on to asepsis, in which efforts are made to prevent bacteria reaching wounds, especially those inseparable from surgery. Surgeons now doff outdoor clothes and don clean apparel, wear special shoes, caps and masks, and they scrub up to make their hands clean and wear rubber gloves. These last were suggested by Thomas Watson (1792–1882) in 1843, before the bacteriological era. But it was William Stewart Halsted (1852–1922) of the Johns Hopkins Hospital who brought them into routine surgical practice. This tale of near conquest of surgical infection came especially with the use of the sulphonamides and the later penicillins, as well as other antibiotics. Again they could be used preoperatively for prevention of contamination of wounds, and they could be used to prevent the growth of bacteria inadvertently introduced into the wound during operations, and finally they could be used to cure infections that had become clinically established. By the careful and intensive use of all these methods the rate of wound infection, which used to be such a scourge and killer, has been reduced to a very small percentage for all operations performed. For a few operations it has been necessary to have a germ-free environment. The expenditure of resources to achieve this is great, but with the passage of time it probably will be seen to be necessary for any operation for the greater safety of the patient. Operations have moved from the kitchen table to the modern operating theatre, but this too in its present form will become out of date and looked on as makeshift.

With pain, bleeding and infection largely overcome, surgery has ranged farther and wider in its scope. Earlier in this book it has been shown how surgery long remained appropriate for the treatment of wounds and lesions on the surface and in the arteries of the limbs (aneurysm). The twentieth century has seen surgery become commonplace beneath the surface in the cavities of the abdomen, chest and head. There were, of course, pioneers who did this much earlier, but theirs were isolated instances. It is the control of pain, bleeding, infection and nutrition that have allowed hundreds and thousands of well-trained surgeons to operate in what once were virtually forbidden areas. Prudence forbade such intervention formerly, since the outcome was almost invariably death. It is not possible here to document the changes that have occurred. They have taken place in every branch of surgery. Almost every organ in the body can be the subject of surgical intervention. The biological nature of the organ may determine how successful or otherwise the surgery may be. But almost every few months sees some overcoming of these problems. For instance only a few decades ago it was often impossible satisfactorily to repair a severed artery. Now such reparative surgery is done every day. Sutures and needles have become finer and less likely to cause clotting at suture lines. Clotting can be controlled by other measures too, so that the vessel will remain patent for the passage of blood. And the eyes of the surgeon have been helped by the use of the operating microscope, so that his field of work is seen much magnified.

It is all these that have led to the sometimes successful replantation of limbs and parts of limbs that have been avulsed or cut off. Yet severed nerves are much more obstinate. They can be sutured and aligned, but function is still a matter of biological chance. They may fail to make muscles contract or to get the skin to feel once more. This depends on biological processes which are partly understood but cannot yet be influenced much.

Many organs can be excised without apparent loss of function for the whole body. There has therefore come the concept of reserves of function. When one of two organs, such as the kidney, are ablated the other will carry on and function is restored wholly, not halved, as might be expected. It is possible to go as far as removing one and a half kidneys without undue detriment to the patient. The same is true of lungs and much of the liver, as well as long lengths of the alimentary tract. But this does not apply to the heart or brain or spinal cord. The differences reside in the biological processes, not the surgical ones. Yet just as the biological processes of many organs have yielded up their secrets in the past, they probably will for these so far intractable ones. This belief is fostered by the recent possibilities of repair. The essential phases of a surgical operation are those of access, of ablation and of repair. To gain access to a part of the body without causing irreparable damage elsewhere is an exploitation of anatomy and this problem has been largely solved. Ablation of a diseased part is similar, but here damage to tissues and organs that are close by has to be avoided for the result may be disastrous. But if the damage can be repaired by one means or another then the extent of ablation can be the maximum necessary for cure.

It is this concept, rarely formally stated, that lies at the back of 'spare-part' surgery. Various organs can be made to serve to replace removed ones. For instance this is done when the oesophagus and stomach are removed and other parts of the intestine are brought in to replace them. Other examples are where skin is taken from a donor site in the same patient to cover over a defect elsewhere; or a segment of vein may be taken from a limb to serve as an arterial conduit in the coronary vessels of the heart; bone is transposed and grafted in many situations. Great ingenuity has been displayed by surgeons using materials at hand in the patient to repair defects caused by disease and its treatment by surgery. But there is a limit to which these local resources can be stretched. A major constraint is occasioned by the necessity for a transposed or grafted organ or tissue to have a blood supply that will maintain its integrity in the new position. This problem can be partly overcome, as it has been, by careful anatomical and surgical studies on blood supplies and the use of arterial and venous anastomoses, using microsurgery when necessary. However, there are still limits to what can yet be done. Better than this sometimes is to obtain materials from elsewhere to function as replacements. This was first done with success in the case of blood, for every transfusion is a form of transplantation using one person's tissues to replace someone else's temporarily. And another successful transplant programme has been that of using donor cornea to replace opacities in the eye with new transparent biological material.

Then there have been repairs effected by the use of man-made materials (physics, chemistry and engineering again). An outstanding example is that of replacement of the osteoarthritic hip joint, causing much pain. A pioneer in this was John Charnley (1911–1982) using shaped plastic and metal and cement in a facsimile of the normal joint. The process is rapidly extending to the knee and ankle and finger joints. Heart valves can be replaced with artificial ones. These in an essential sense are all relatively simple mechanical substitutes, but some structures have highly complex functions which cannot be so simply replaced. Then the only recourse is to use whole donor organs.

Any reader of the public press, or viewer of television, knows that transplantation of organs from the dying or the dead is now done extensively. Kidney transplantation is probably the most successful, but the liver, pancreas (for diabetes), heart and lungs are all slowly yielding to technological advances. There is an essential simplicity about the surgery in excising the diseased organs and connecting up the new donor organ by its blood vessels and ducts. To do the job demands immense knowledge, skill, patience and stamina but the underlying concept is not difficult. The real problem is that of rejection of the donated organ or tissue, and this is the result of immunological responses. Personal bodily identity is maintained by a variety of mechanisms, some of which have been mentioned earlier. Foreign material of almost any kind is recognized and efforts are made to reject it. This is biologically right in all normal situations, but becomes inappropriate and damaging in such surgical interventions. It is the understanding of the immunological rejection processes in a very artificial situation, together with its pharmacological and biological suppression, that have made transplant surgery possible on a now large scale. When Christiaan Barnard (1922–) in Cape Town reported on his first cardiac transplant in 1967 it was received as a breakthrough by the public press. Medically there was greater doubt since it was known that though the operation was obviously technically feasible and had been for many years, the immunological problems seemed to have been largely ignored. There are always those who counsel waiting until more knowledge has come in, and those who wish to get ahead, seeing obstacles in greater simplicity than the objectors. Whatever else the results of Barnard's experiment have been it led to many more researches into immune mechanisms, so that almost daily the transplantation of organs becomes safer and more successful. Without the efforts and actions of many pioneers and their patients, willing to take a risk, little progress in this form of surgery would have been made.

In an historical context this is not a new departure. At the start every procedure carries risk. Only continuing experiment will show whether the risks are worth running, or if they can be reduced by acceptable levels. Acceptance is cultural (both medical and general), not statistical or scientific. This is where the non-medical public has its rights to be heard. It is the public that determines the cultural values within which medicine and surgery are practised. The fact that those values may often be emotional, inexact and prejudiced does not alter the other fact that the medical profession acts under 'licence', vaguely defined, granted by the culture in which it operates. When that licence appears to be too constrictive it is up to the profession by persuasion to change the cultural values. These will vary from country to country, and from group to group in each society. Conflicts of values between medicine and society need a better forum for discussion than they have so far had.

The triumphs of surgery, based as they are in many other disciplines and subjects, have rubbed off into gynaecology. At the turn of the century venereal diseases split away from it. It then became a mainly surgical subject dealing with cancers and other large tumours, as well as controlling haemorrhage by surgical means in ectopic pregnancies and spontaneous abortions, and also in repair of uterovaginal prolapse, then so common among relatively undernourished poor women, who were hard working and also producing many children. In 1902 Ernst Wertheim (1864–1920) in Vienna introduced his radical operation for the treatment of cervical cancer. Despite the vaginal operation for the same condition brought in by Friedrich Schauta (1849–1919), also of Vienna, the Wertheim operation held the field, until recently. Its recession was due to the improvement in radiotherapy which offers just as good results, but with less mortality and less morbidity than operation. This exemplifies a general trend to be observed in all branches of surgery. Just as an operation becomes established some other, more medical less invasive, therapy begins to displace it. There is a natural feeling on all sides that surgery is to be avoided whenever possible. Even now radiotherapy is being overtaken by chemotherapy in the treatment of many malignant tumours. When the treatments have been perfected for more and more cancers there will be less and less need for the relative crudities of radical surgery. Surgery will then become more rational in dealing with the mechanical problems of trauma and the unblocking of vital tubes that have been obstructed by tumours. At base cancer is a biological or biochemical process. It will yield to physical and chemical therapies ultimately for they are more fundamental than those of surgery.

Prolapse is an anatomical problem, in which the supports of the uterus, vagina and pelvic organs are weakened. The surgical treatment of the condition is mechanical and therefore rational. It began with Archibald Donald's (1860–1937) operation in 1908 devised in Manchester, England, where patients were often impoverished mill-hands. It was publicized and modified by William Edward Fothergill (1865–1926) of the same city in 1915. With further modifications it became the Manchester operation, though throughout the world others were proceeding on similar lines and attached different names to what they were doing.

The real advance of the twentieth century was, however, in understanding the physiology and pathology of the uterine (menstrual) cycles and their dependence on ovarian cycles, all being part of the general development of endocrinology. It had long been known that if the ovaries were removed then menstruation ceased. Understanding how this was brought about depended on the isolation of oestrin from the ovaries in 1923 by Edgar Allen (1892–1943) and Edward Adelbert Doisy (1893–). This was shown to be a hormone, as was progesterone, the other main secretion of the ovary, characterized by George Washington Corner (1889–1981) and Willard Myron Allen (1904–) in 1929. Shortly after it was shown how these two substances affected the endometrium (lining of the uterus) to bring about changes there resulting finally in menstruation. Prior to this time the changes were virtually inexplicable, though they had been described, and often were attributed to inflammation. The new knowledge wrought immense changes in the practice of gynaecology since the hormones were used in practice to control menstrual disorders, from which almost every woman suffers at some time in her reproductive lifetime. Then came Gregory Goodwin Pincus (1903–1967), who in 1953 showed that progesterone would suppress ovulation in the rabbit. He was soon to develop oral contraception in humans based on this discovery.

The method is now in use by millions of women throughout the world and may well have been instrumental in changing sexual mores in many societies, a matter still much debated. Of course the whole idea of contraception was creeping into society's acceptances in the first few decades of the twentieth century. It was pushed forward by such as Marie Stopes (1880–1928) and it was also vigorously resisted on moral and other grounds. In her time there were only the methods of the safe period (so-called), of withdrawal, of the condom and a variety of diaphragms for insertion into the vagina. There had also been introduced the metal ring of Ernst Grafenberg (1881–1957) in 1926 in which the object was inserted into the uterine cavity to prevent embedding of the fertilized ovum. It has achieved some popularity in use only in the past two decades as the intrauterine contraceptive device. This became possible because of new plastic and metal developments which diminished the side-effects of having a foreign body more or less permanently in place in the uterus. But the oral combined (oestrogen + progesterone) contraceptive pill revolutionized ideas about contraception and has become quite the most popular method nowadays in advanced and educated societies. There are still drawbacks to the use of the pill, but as they come to light they tend to be overcome or much decreased.

Infections of the genital tract used to wreak much havoc in causing infertility by gonorrhoea and in affecting fetuses and children by syphilis. These have been only partially controlled by penicillin and other antibiotics, the success being much less with gonorrhoea than with syphilis. This may in part be due to the certain increase that there has been in sexual promiscuity since sexual intercourse has been separated from its common aftermath of pregnancy by the reliable birth control method of the pill. But another main factor has been the emergence of strains of gonococci that have grown resistant to each antibiotic in turn. These bacteria seem able to do this because of their genetic make-up which allows them to adapt to the inimical environment to which they are exposed when antibiotic therapy is used extensively. The control of these major infections (incomplete though it is) has brought to light a whole new range of sexually transmitted diseases, of the vagina and the pelvic female organs. The most important are some viruses and chlamydia. There will never be any peace from infections nor any in the constant search for agents to combat them. This has become manifest for all organs and tissues. It is a condition of life. Microbes of all kinds have a will to live and so adapt and re-adapt to all the slings and arrows launched against them. This is Darwinian evolution in daily action, based on the processes of genetic variation acted on by factors in the environment.

Cervical cancer is a relatively common disease and the cervix is accessible to inspection and biopsy through short vaginal specula. This has made the organ of value in understanding some of the processes of neoplasia in general. In particular it was found possible to scrape superficial cells off the cervix with a simple wooden spatula. After fixing and staining the cells are visible under the microscope, and this has brought about the new specialty of cytology, concerned with the morphology of cells. Also the cervix can have small biopsy samples removed from it so that cytological appearances can be easily correlated with histological ones. This has been much used in diagnosis, but more importantly in the long term it has shed light on the natural history of cancer in general. There is first a cellular change which may regress, but if it progresses then cancer cells grow but at first do not penetrate into underlying tissues. It is such penetration that is characteristic of cancer, but before taking on this property of invasion there may be a long latent interval of up to 10 or 15 years. The concept is exciting since it raises the possibilities of prevention of the later invasive and killing phases of cancer in many sites. The process has begun somewhat crudely in gynaecology, where if by smears and biopsy a non-invasive lesion is found it may be excised locally by scalpel or cautery, or indeed the whole uterus including the cervix may be removed. But matters are going beyond this since the introduction of the colposcope which is an optical instrument by which the cervix can be seen much magnified, and areas of abnormal epithelium and blood vessels can be visualized. Diagnosis is then more precise and the abnormal area may be destroyed by laser beam. This avoids minor or major surgery, which was all that was available at first, and avoids too the sometimes unpleasant side-effects of surgery.

Again this ease of access to the cervix has led to understanding of the possible part played by virus infections in the genesis of cancer. This may have more general applicability. It has long been suspected that the first change to make a cell cancerous resides in its genetic constitution. It now appears that such a change may be occasioned by a virus, perhaps like the herpes virus which is commonly found in the female genital tract. The process of cancer is therefore being unravelled. There is the obvious analogy with the earlier analysis of chemical metabolic processes, dependent on physical and chemical technology. Now that biology has developed its own sophisticated techniques, biochemical, genetic and cellular chains of development will become increasingly clear. Just as with metabolic chains it will become possible to intervene purposefully in the biological ones to re-direct them towards normality. The question hanging over this progress is not whether it will happen, but when. The inventiveness is already there, but it needs money and resources, with political will, to give it reign.

Gynaecology has also found techniques for the treatment of infertility and subfertility, especially in forcing ovulation to occur by endocrine treatment, and in surgery on blockages in the Fallopian tubes, sometimes using microsurgical instruments. The world was startled in the 1970s to find that Patrick Steptoe and R. G. Edwards in England had been able to obtain ova and fertilize them in the laboratory so that they would grow and could then be inserted into the uterus to produce a normal baby. This brought the usual anxieties about morality and whether it was right to do this. The other operations of gynaecology in sterilizing women, and in performing abortions on them raised similar worries. Matters of reproduction and interference with them in the directions of promotion or prevention touch the conscience of all societies deeply. Culture then begins to make itself felt in the concerns of medicine. It is now an important interface, shown especially in gynaecology, but also in some transplantations, especially those for the heart—also an organ about which society feels deeply. Yet all these new techniques are a natural historical progression from what has gone before. They are no different in essence from previously. This has been touched on in the earlier consideration of transplants in this book. As regards gynaecology every community has had an abiding interest in the promotion of fertility and at the same time prevention of births in individuals.

There is the well-known allusion to Egyptian camel-drivers some thousands of years BC who put pebbles into the uteri of their female beasts to prevent them calving, and now we have the plastic intrauterine device, the very notion of which upsets some people. Every new technique in these popularly sensitive areas of human life causes a readjustment in cultural thinking. But always in the past culture has assimilated them and adapted itself. In time these present moral problems will dissolve, become accepted and be replaced by others.

Obstetrics began this century with the introduction of antenatal care by John William Ballantyne (1861–1923) of Edinburgh, in 1902. He had two in-patient beds for pregnant patients. One of his major aims was the understanding and prevention of congenital defects in babies. This did not become practicable until Gregg, in 1940 in Australia, made his discoveries of rubella in pregnancy as a cause of blindness, deafness and heart disease in the young. The idea of antenatal care was quickly taken up in the USA in Boston, and in Adelaide in Australia, and ultimately, in one form or another, throughout the world. The aim partly switched to the early recognition and prevention of disease and disorder in the mother both in pregnancy and labour. The results appeared to be spectacular because of the steady decline in maternal deaths that occurred. In England and Wales in 1928 the maternal mortality rate was 4.42 per 1000 births. By 1975 it had dropped to 0.11 per 1000 (excluding abortions). However, antenatal care is only one of several factors influencing the fall. Perhaps the most significant may be the increasing height and weight of women over the decades as a result of improved nutrition in childhood, and better hygiene which prevented some infectious diseases apt to injure girls' health and later make them relatively unfit to bear children themselves. Taller women, with a weight commensurate for their height, in general have a much better prognosis for bearing healthy children and rearing them than others less well endowed physically, economically and socially. Smaller families as a result of wider use of contraception seem to have made it possible for greater parental care to be lavished on the few rather than be spread among many. Childbearing women have, by natural processes, become better able to withstand the problems that might beset them in pregnancy, labour, puerperium and the early years of their babies' childhoods.

The techniques of obstetrics have improved too. The pharmacological revolution earlier referred to has made it possible to treat such potential killers of mothers and babies as diabetes, heart disease and kidney disease. Pre-eclamptic toxaemia, a potentially serious complication specific to childbearing women, has become largely preventable and sometimes treatable by drugs. But the most dramatic change has been the control and treatment of infection and of haemorrhage at many points in the process of childbearing. Prior to about the middle of the twentieth century these groups of disorders must have carried off millions of women in their prime. Now their effects are infinitesimal as compared with formerly, and by comparison with the 100 million or so births that occur throughout the world annually. It will be seen that obstetrics has adapted general advances in medicine and surgery for its own more specific ends.

Techniques have been developed in obstetrics that are more directed to its own problems, such as those of delivery. Christian Kielland (1871–1941) of Oslo produced a new design of obstetric forceps in 1916. They solved the problem of the fetal head being stuck in a transverse position in labour by allowing it to be rotated with the forceps actually in position on the head. The older types of forceps, if used in this way, caused untold damage. Many other types of forceps have been invented during the twentieth century, one of the more popular being the small ones of Arthur Joseph Wrigley (1902–1984), brought out in 1936. They were valuable for the use of general practitioners who at that time conducted many deliveries in homes and nursing homes, before hospitals became the usual place for delivery. It is a sign of the times that this change in birth practice has happened—another exemplification of the fact that all branches of medicine have become specialized. And, of course, the operations of obstetrics—particularly caesarean section—have become safer both for mothers and for babies because of the advances in anaesthesia, transfusion and treatment of infection, all of which have so vitally influenced the development of surgery. Problems that have arisen in labour over the centuries can now be side-stepped completely by performing caesarean section. In up to 10 per cent of births in advanced countries this is how delivery is effected.

The uterus in labour (and indeed throughout reproductive life) behaves differently from any other form of muscle in its contractions. Now these can be more or less controlled by increasing them with a drip of the hormone, oxytocin, found by Dale and used in obstetrics by William Blair-Bell (1871–1936) of Liverpool in 1909. There have been many refinements and changes since these early days. And John Chassar Moir (1900–1977) refined ergot, which had been known for centuries, and characterized ergometrine. This is in world-wide use to prevent post-partum haemorrhage. Although the prostaglandins are not so universally used it is worth remembering that they were first discovered by seminal fluid being put into the uterus and observing the contractions thus caused. These substances are now known to be widespread in the body and in their actions, forming part of the understanding of cellular biology.

It is impossible to separate the practice of obstetrics from the care of the newborn and that of the fetus *in utero*. For a long time there was comparatively little that could be done about either of them, nature having to be left to take its course. There was always the hope that if the mother were brought to childbed safe and healthy, then there would be a spin-off for the baby. First came better understanding of the physiology of the newborn and how it differed from that of the adult. The establishment of breathing was an important aspect of this. The already noted advances in control of infection, of haemorrhage and the introduction of some of the techniques of the anaesthetist helped to make the first few hours of life safer. Water and mineral metabolism came to be understood, so that surgery for the correction of abnormalities in tiny babies was possible and practised. The causes of the various anomalies of development are slowly becoming known too, so that prevention has become at least a possibility. This led to attempts to investigate directly the state of the fetus *in utero*. Crudely, if an abnormality can be found early enough, then the pregnancy can be terminated by abortion. The hope for the future is that something more refined than this can be found to bring about correction of anomalies.

Some serious disorders are linked with the sex of the child. In 1949 Murray Llewellyn Barr (1908–) and Ewart George Bartram (1923–) showed that every cell could be characterized as either male or female by the presence of a small piece of chromatin present at the edge of the nucleus in all female cells, yet absent from male ones. Fetuses shed cells from their epithelia into the amniotic fluid surrounding them. A needle inserted through the abdominal wall into the fluid can withdraw samples for examination. If a fetus is male (say) in a family liable to have a sex-linked disorder then the fetus can be aborted. Various enzymatic disorders can be demonstrated in similar fashion and the same 'remedy' applied. It was in obstetrics too that Ian Donald (1910–) first applied ultrasonics to investigate the fetus and early embryo by an imaging technique that was non-invasive and safe. This has been much enlarged in scope since his description of 1961 and has come largely to replace X-rays used in pregnancy which are potentially damaging to the embryo and fetus. And the technique has been and is continuing to be applied to many other areas of the body. Attempts are being made too to introduce viewing instruments safely into the amniotic cavity so that the fetus and placenta can be directly inspected. The functions of the placenta (afterbirth) on which the fetus depends so heavily are being investigated by biochemical and endocrine methods with a view to recognizing when its life-support systems are failing so that the baby can be delivered before it is impaired.

These examples from obstetrics and gynaecology are taken because these are the subjects in which the author has spent a professional lifetime and also because they exemplify in general terms what has happened in other disciplines. Medicine is indivisible despite the necessary increasing specialization. Ideas and techniques are forever ebbing and flowing across the boundaries, being taken up, discarded and adapted to meet the special needs of each subject and how its problems are being viewed by its practitioners at any particular time. The significance of the problems is determined by day-to-day practice where they arise from within the discipline so that, by many means of communication, groups begin to try to solve them. In this they draw on ideas and techniques belonging to the general body of medicine and surgery, and in time what is being done is subject to the scrutiny of the general public. Their views too help to determine significance.

As a result of what has been outlined above there has grown the specialty of neonatology. Some paediatricians devote all or a major part of their time to newborn babies, and some surgeons do too. Since obstetricians have specialized in the problems of the fetus as distinct from the mother and the newborn, there has to be teamwork between paediatrician, obstetrician and neonatal surgeon, and this new discipline has become known as perinatology. In this century the specialty of paediatrics, dealing with the problems of children, has undergone major changes. In the earlier years there were problems of malnutrition, even starvation, and infection of many kinds, especially respiratory and bone and joint tuberculosis. There were all the epidemic diseases and their aftermaths, with measles, whooping cough and gastroenteritis claiming their victims. All are still present though in much less degree. This has come about by understanding natural history, allowing of prevention sometimes, but especially because of immunization programmes and the coming of antibiotics and chemotherapy. The fact that many of these measures have become commonplace does not diminish the necessity for continuing vigilance and much routine hard work by an army of those in health care. As these numerically large problems have come under some sort of control other disorders have come into prominence—especially congenital abnormalities and inborn errors of metabolism and growth, as well as endocrine disorders and malignant tumours of all kinds.

Perhaps the outstanding development in the twentieth century in the intellectual world has been that of psychology and psychiatry. It pervades all medical practice (or it should) and also that of personal and social relationships, the arts and sciences, and indeed everything where people are in communication with one another, verbally or non-verbally. Few can now resist the interpretation of themselves or others in psychological, and even psychiatric, terms. This was less likely when life was nasty, brutish and short, beset by economic, military, medical, nutritional, physical, hygienic and other environmental vicissitudes. As these have relatively diminished, attention has been directed to mental and social life. The changed physical conditions of life allied with new theories and demonstrations of the mental ones have made this possible. Concern with psychology can come about only when life in general is physically more comfortable and some of the old physical and biological human enemies are held in some degree of check.

There had been tentative probings into the subject of psychiatry in the eighteenth and nineteenth centuries. In 1883 Emil Kraepelin (1856–1926) wrote his *Compendium der Psychiatrie* delineating many mental disorders. Three years later Richard von Krafft-Ebing (1840–1902) wrote *Psychopathia Sexualis*. Between 1900 and 1928 Henry Havelock Ellis (1859–1939) produced the seven volumes of his *Studies in the Psychology of Sex*. In rapid succession were Sigmund Freud (1856–1939) on psychopathology in 1904, Alfred Adler (1870–1937) in 1907 on some aspects of neurosis and Carl Gustav Jung (1875–1961) on psychoanalysis and his interpretations of analytical psychology in 1912. Pierre Marie Félix Janet (1859–1947) in 1923 wrote on *La Médecine Psychologique*, introducing useful ideas about hysteria. The world of psychological medicine was very much astir in the first quarter of the twentieth century. Some of the views expounded, particularly those to do with sexuality and dissecting minds by psychoanalysis, were shocking to the general conscience. It is interesting to compare this opposition with that to the start of anatomy in the sixteenth century and earlier.

It is surely not necessary to emphasize how psychology and psychiatry have flourished since these early decades of the twentieth century. In medicine these disciplines undertake the treatment of more patients than almost all of the other specialties together. The subject has split into several disciplines—those of adult psychiatry, child and adolescent psychiatry, mental handicap, psychogeriatrics, forensic psychiatry and psychosexual medicine. All are now specialties requiring experts, trained over long periods for each job, whereas earlier one person could cope with all of them. The patterns of such specialization are familiar enough.

The drug revolution of the second half of the century has brought in chemical treatments for many of the neuroses. Psychoses and psychopathic personalities are at present much more resistant to such help. Their fundamental pathology is not well understood in the biological/chemical mode.

Mental handicap too gives rise to immense difficulties, though light has been shed on some of the disorders by knowledge of inborn errors of metabolism, and by the discovery of a genetic basis for Down's syndrome by Lionel Sharples Penrose (1898–1972), and subsequently in other abnormalities. In some of these studies lies the possibility of prevention of mental handicap, and also the opportunity to reduce the total amount of it by selective abortion.

The physical approach to the treatment of mental disorder has been seen in psychosurgery, in which parts of the brain are cut through, and in electroconvulsive therapy. These have run into much opposition both within the ranks of the psychiatrists and those outside. The drugs are tending to supersede the physical approaches, along with other forms of psychotherapy. There is a tension between those who see the brain and mind as very complex chemical mechanisms, amenable therefore to forms of chemical therapy, and those who see the mind as a partially separate entity from the brain, and therefore amenable to psychological therapies. In the present state of knowledge both attitudes are sustainable and tenable without serious refutation of one by the other. In fact most psychiatrists are pragmatists, using the tools to hand for their patients, whether the methods are in essence chemical or psychological. Very few hold entrenched positions on this essentially philosophical problem, stemming from the dualism of mind and body argued for by Descartes in the seventeenth century.

Generally more important than these specific subjects of psychiatry has been the diffusion of attitudes about psychology and psychiatry into all medical practice and into many other areas of life and society. In the best medicine the effect of any physical disorder in the patient on his intellectual and emotional functioning, of the mind on the disease process and of the role of the mind in causing physical disorder are all taken into account in order better to help the patient or client cope with his problems. Whereas diagnosis was once made in purely physical, pathological terms, it now includes a psychological component.

The growth of psychology, with its especial consideration of personal relationships, has furthered the development of sociology in its studies of the relationships of groups of people, in a variety of situations. The behaviour of groups is determined by the psychology of those individuals that make them up. It is not intended to delve into the ramifications of the social sciences, but they too have had their effects on medicine. A patient may become ill because of his social relationships with which he may not be in harmony. These affect his psychology (perhaps emerging into a psychiatric malady) and this reacts on those in his immediate surroundings, particularly members of his family and in his workplace. He may, as a result, become physically ill. And in the reverse direction a person who is ill physically shows a psychological reaction to his illness, and in its turn this affects the reactions of his family, his neighbours, and those with whom he works.

This nexus of relationships is complex and also needs consideration in establishing a full diagnosis of a particular patient's problems. A diagnosis therefore has physical, psychological and social components. At different times and in different patients varying significances have to be placed on these factors. Inevitably, general practitioners will have a major interest in the psychology and sociology of their patients, as will psychologists and sociologists; and those in hospital practice will more greatly emphasize the physical aspects of patients' illnesses. But it is not to be assumed that these generalists and specialists concentrate *only* on one factor or another. This is a criticism often voiced and it is fallacious from the start. It is partly a result of the misreading of the significance of specialization which we have seen is inseparable from the history of the twentieth century.

The story of specialization in the twentieth century could be extended *ad nauseam*, but for this book that would be to no purpose. Depending on how categories are defined there are about 55 specialties now recognized within medical practice. There is no wonder that it cannot be encompassed fully by any single mind, whereas in previous centuries it was at least thought to be possible. Practitioners then often held themselves out as capable of managing all known diseases, in diagnosis, prognosis and treatment. They were indeed general practitioners in medicine, surgery, midwifery and therapeutics. No one would now dare to claim such omnicompetence, in both knowledge and skills. The response to all this specialization could only be what it has been—teamwork. It may be that a patient consults only one person in the first instance, but then, as the case demands, the doctor calls into play one and then another. And the specialization has gone far beyond the confines of the medical profession. There have to be medical secretaries, filing clerks, administrators, finance officers, caterers, launderers, maintenance staff, porters, nurses, physiotherapists, occupational therapists, radiographers, midwives, physicists, chemists, psychologists, electronic engineers, operating theatre technicians and many others, all specialists and skilled in their own ways. Directly and indirectly they are all part of the team which cares for and attempts to help the patient or client with his or her maladies.

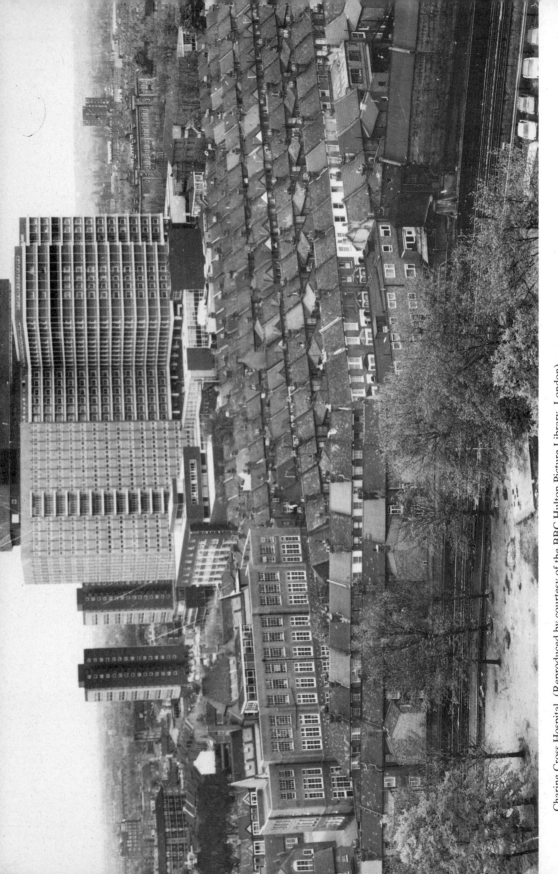

Charing Cross Hospital. (Reproduced by courtesy of the BBC Hulton Picture Library, London)

Chapter 11

Medicine and society

The specializations within medicine and its increasing complexity have demanded responses from within the profession, arising out of its own progress in knowledge and skills, and from outside because of society's proper concern with what is being done for it in the name of medicine. The medical organization is one arm of society's endeavours to look after its own members. When sickness strikes there is a moral obligation, deeply felt, to provide succour. Once this was incumbent upon family, friends, neighbours and tribe. Then the obligation extended to cities and nations as civilization advanced. The responses of society to these felt needs may be partially traced in the growth of institutions. Institutions are bodies of people set up as organizations designed to meet a need, which may not at first be obvious to the general public, but by the activities of the institutions its attention may be directed towards satisfying that need. This is the way in which charities become directed to some specific ends, and as public opinion about those ends gathers strength then the State may have to take political notice. The general process may be illustrated by medical examples.

The hospitals of antiquity in Greek, Egyptian and Roman times (in Cos, Alexandria, Salerno and on the Tiber) show some social concern for the plight of the suffering. It is an early glimmer, brightening for a while and then being extinguished. For aeons, however, the norm of medical care seems to have been that of the family or slightly larger group looking after its sick members in a received traditional amateur fashion. In desperate personal straits magicians, sorcerers, charlatans, quacks, wise-women, necromancers, soothsayers, herbalists and physicians and surgeons might be called in to help in return for some form of payment.

The distinction of the amateur from the professional was very blurred, and indeed was scarcely made. The doctors partook of many of the characteristics of their rivals and employed some of their techniques. There are cynics who believe that they still do! There is some truth in the charge for many people wish for their doctors to be miracle workers, and it is flattering to the profession when it seems that a wonderful, almost supernatural, cure has been effected in a case where everything appeared to be hopeless. The reactions on both sides are usual enough. They satisfy some sort of human need. It would be foolish of any healer to ignore them, though he or she might also be wise not to arrogate to himself or herself too much of the credit that should be accorded to nature—the *vis medicatrix naturae*.

The power of mind, emotion and faith in the bringing about of cures both in physical and in mental disorders, or of making patients feel better in distressing disease, are not to be gainsaid. Consciously or unconsciously they enter into all healing relationships. No doctor ignores them; he even uses them, though he may realize that their place in healing is not yet scientifically proved.

It is still insufficiently understood that thoughtful doctors do not dismiss these intangibles from their practice, nor do they say that their patients do not feel better sometimes after consulting practitioners outside the medical profession. The doctors, however, do seek to quantify the results of alternative therapies and evaluate them against their own medical practices. They want to know how and to what extent these alternative therapies work. The results might then become more public and more widely used because they would then have a basis that could be scientifically tested. So far many alternative therapies are unable to produce this basis. The evidence in their favour is anecdotal. That does not make it untrue, only for the present unverifiable or falsifiable. This does not make for condemnation, but only for suspension of judgement. This last is rare and its lack is shown throughout much of normal everyday medical practice too. Many presently accepted scientifically based practices arose in the distant past from the sorts of trials that present alternative therapies carry on now. But, as with many other such trials, only time will bring evidence to show whether they have a lasting place in medicine or not. New ideas can sink into oblivion as well as flourish.

In the centuries around AD 1000 many hospitals were founded throughout Europe, and especially in London, mainly in association with monastic foundations. They were often hospices for pilgrims, and for the indigent in their neighbourhoods. Inevitably there was some increase in professionalism of those who worked in the wards. Also, somewhat later, many cities, especially in Germany, appointed town physicians and midwives to help to look after citizens and to advise the authorities on matters of public health. But all these were relatively isolated instances, though they show the dawning of some social ideas concerning medicine and medical and health care. Then in 1518 in London the College of Physicians was founded with a charter from Henry VIII. This was essentially a move by which physicians could distance themselves from the 'lesser breeds without the law', such as surgeons and apothecaries. The intention was to identify themselves as a special group controlling practice within 7 miles of the City of London, supervising the practice of other practitioners and determining entry standards to the profession of physicianship.

It was largely protective of the physicians, yet it contained a germ of an idea in the control of standards which has mightily borne fruit in subsequent centuries. In retrospect the standards of the time were ludicrous, in that only graduates of Oxford and Cambridge Universities were eligible to be members of the College, and they had to pass an oral examination of about 20 minutes' duration which was conducted in Latin. This was intended to show whether the candidate had an adequate knowledge of the ancient masters of medicine. Such physicians had essentially to be educated gentlemen of the times, fit to supervise surgeons and apothecaries and to oversee the quality of drugs bought from the apothecaries' shops. Nevertheless a standard was established for entry and that standard was formally assessed. These two processes have been the foundation of medical education since. They were known in the mediaeval universities and perhaps even as far back as Plato's Academy, but they were not widely acknowledged before the time of the College of Physicians in medicine. Entry to the trades of barber–surgeon and apothecary was through serving an apprenticeship. It is the uniting of supervised experience with the setting of standards of entry and the assessment of these for each individual candidate that have become the norm for medical education in the western world. There has been much development of these ideas in detail but the principles are still there and are more ancient than is usually realized.

By 1540 there was founded the Company of Barber–Surgeons in London, which was a craft guild. To enter the Company an apprentice had to serve a master until he became a journeyman and ultimately a master himself. The elements of this are still to be seen in medical education, where at first responsibility exercised by the student is slight and supervision of work is close, and as time passes responsibility is increased and supervision lessens. It took till 1617 before the Society of Apothecaries was founded, and by then the tripartite profession—consisting of physicians, surgeons and apothecaries—was more or less established. This is not to say that this had occurred fully nation-wide. But it slowly diffused from the centre in London, and from other capital cities throughout Europe so that this arrangement has become almost universal. Apothecaries used to have shops, but they also gave medical advice, and they have become general practitioners. For a long time the surgeons and apothecaries worked under the general supervision of physicians, but increasing professionalism and specialization have cast off this yoke. This came about gradually for the surgeons when they first split off from the Barbers as the Company of Surgeons in 1745 and later when they became the Royal College of Surgeons of England in 1800. The Royal College of General Practitioners did not finally emerge until 1952.

Although the Colleges might be seen now as being set up to advance the causes of the professions, it is also true that they were in some measure responding to inarticulate needs of the public and various governing authorities. At least there were identifiable groups or corporate bodies representative of some professional interests on which political pressures of one kind and another could be brought to bear. And from Parliament and other institutions there was a channel along which needs and requirements could be made known. The stage was being set for dialogue between profession and public. It was perhaps not fully recognized at the time, but that is how it has turned out. The dialogue is still faltering and embryonic, but the mechanisms for its conduct are there and can be further developed, as they are being.

There had, of course, been some organization of medicine to meet specific needs in the navy and the army. Some inkling of these has been given earlier and there is no room to expand the topic in detail. But it is out of these military (and other) arrangements that there came ideas about the importance of the environment in which work (albeit military and naval) is done and of diseases apt to affect those in certain occupations. This has led to the specializations of occupational health and of the whole public health movement of the nineteenth century especially. This has expanded further into what is now known as community medicine or community health, which has been described as looking at the 'population as a patient'. It has been a major development of the last few decades in which groups of people are seen and investigated in their total environments. The specialty has been fed by morsels taken from public health, sanitation, housing, nutrition, growth, sociology, statistics, physiology, ergonomics, administrative and management theory and many other disciplines. It is a specialized part of ideas paralleled in sociology and in biology. Those who wish to investigate society in one of its myriad parameters and those who market and sell goods and services all look for characteristics of groups that they can express in statistical terms, and medicine has to do the same in order to function as an arm of society, which now not only has a concern for its individual members but also for the contexts in which they have their being.

The problem of community medicine, as of occupational medicine, is that having found out facts about groups of people, those facts have to be pressed on those in authority so that action on those facts and ideas generated by them may be taken. It is here that medicine is particularly to be seen as acting on and being acted on by society in general. A clinical doctor can initiate action on and with individuals. A community doctor or one in occupational health has to try to mobilize social action, which is much more diffuse and difficult, for it requires persuasion of others to act on behalf of a community. Results and end-points are then nearly impossible to gauge and cannot be as clear cut as they are clinically. This explains much of the disaffection of community physicians who seek a role that is credible for themselves; within the rest of the medical profession; among other professionals in similar fields; and with lay persons in authority who have it in their power either to act or not to act on the advice that they receive. The interface between medicine and society is most clearly visible here, and shows how society ultimately controls medicine and medical practice. This bridle often chafes, for the medical profession has not yet been broken to accept it. Nor will it, for in a democracy there must be continuing dialogue, argument and discussion. The medical profession has its rights to argue and so does society, and each must be prepared for continuing debate, often heated. There cannot be, nor should there be, any final rapprochement. Constraints and pressures must be exerted by both sides. There is no other way. Realization of this can reduce anger and frustration, neither of which is helpful nor productive.

The wholesale incursion of society into the affairs of medicine began with the passing of the Medical Act of 1858. Similar governmental moves were made about the same time in many other countries than the United Kingdom. Before the Act went through Parliament there had been many other attempts to get bills passed. Obviously there were anxieties in the minds of doctors and legislators that medicine should come under more control than had previously been exercised. There was recognition that the medical profession ought to be better organized than it had been so that it could more properly serve the public for whose interest it was supposed to work. The method to be used to do this was by the control of medical education. It deserves to be noted that practice itself was not amenable to control; but it was assumed, and still is, that if education is controlled then standards of practice can be maintained at a level that is satisfactory for the public.

In the event the General Medical Council was set up. Its main tool of authority was the Medical Register which it was and is required to keep. This is a list of names of people by which the public and the profession can distinguish those who are duly medically qualified from those who are not. That, of course, begs the question of how to determine what 'qualified' means. About the middle of the nineteenth century this was not easy in detail. But the principles, ever after accepted not only in the UK but also independently throughout the western world, have emerged. A statutory body (in the UK the GMC but elsewhere possibly a government or State ministry) is set up with authority to prescribe the subjects that shall be studied by an intending qualified doctor; to prescribe the places and institutions in which he or she may study those subjects; to inspect the premises and the staff who give instruction; to determine the general form of examinations and assessments of students and inspect them; and to keep a register of those who have fulfilled all these requirements.

It is the register that holds the final power. The staff, the institutions, and above all the students who comply with the directives laid down by authority may have names registered. If they do not comply then the students cannot become duly qualified doctors. They must conform if they wish for this accolade, which all students desire. The minimum standards for entry to the medical profession are then reasonably assured, and they are constantly monitored by the authoritative body. This has to be essentially made up of doctors, for in any profession it is only the profession that knows and can enforce the standards required of it. Nevertheless, the profession's body is subject to some over-riding control by government. At the very least it is subject to government and political criticism and there is an identifiable body at which that criticism can be levelled. That is part of the dialogue that must go on between society at large and its constituent groups, whatever their nature.

There are variations in detail on this general theme in different countries with their variant cultures and political systems. But every country is concerned with the standards of medical care practised within its jurisdiction and develops mechanisms to ensure that those standards are kept to. The sanctions that may be exerted against any backsliding practitioner may then be criminal or civil action, professional action—in which a doctor may be suspended from practice either temporarily or permanently, when his name is removed from the Medical Register—or both. This sort of control is generally used for all professions, some trades and crafts, and in different countries and cultures, with variation in detail and with differing degrees of efficacy. Medicine seems to have progressed further along this road than many others because of its long history, its developed traditions, its developed system of ethical behaviour and the increasingly overt concern of the public in medical affairs. Medicine is increasingly seen to belong to the public and not to the profession. It has always been so but is now more obvious than it used to be.

The first Medical Act of 1858 brought the providers of medical education under central control. These were mainly the universities and medical schools, some of which were private. The growth of a bureaucratic society has meant the discontinuance of private medical education separated from the universities in most places in the western world. Medicine and medical education have become too important for society and government to allow them to be essentially entrepreneurial and without checks. Interestingly this means that universities are far from autonomous in controlling the medical curriculum. This is imposed on them by an outside professional body. In the UK this is the GMC which is in constant dialogue with organs of government. Other non-medical professional disciplines taught in universities also come under similar constraints, but not perhaps as extensively as in medicine. It is only in certain non-professional subjects that the universities entirely set their curricula and standards in a formal way, not greatly subject to outside inspection.

Since 1858 there have been many amending Medical Acts as the relationships within medicine and between it and society have changed. These are matters of detail outside the present scope. And not only this but other professions of medical care have pursued the same directions. An Act of 1902 set up the Central Midwives Board exactly analogous to that for doctors to control the educational standards, entry to practice and the keeping of a register for midwives so that midwifery might become more professionalized. In the twentieth century too came the General Nursing Council in 1946 (now re-vamped again) and the Council for Professions Supplementary to Medicine later. It can be seen how each profession follows similar courses, and again the process is inexorably world-wide with some countries progressing more rapidly than others. All of these are institutional responses to needs felt within the increasingly specialized professions and outside them in the general organs of society and its actions.

Within medicine the adolescence or coming of age of many of the specialties, noted in earlier chapters, has been marked by the founding of some Royal Colleges or specialist Faculties within the older Royal Colleges. In 1927 came the present Royal College of Obstetricians and Gynaecologists. From about 1950 onwards there have been Royal Colleges of General Practitioners, of Pathologists, of Psychiatrists, of Radiologists, and numerous Faculties springing up within the Royal Colleges of Physicians and of Surgeons. This fissile reproduction has occurred because groups of specialists have come to feel that they needed separate identity within the total medical profession, which in the mass could not represent their professional needs. The result has been that each College and Faculty has set up its own curricula, its own prescribed experience, its own inspections of places where that experience may be gained, its own examination and assessments and its own distinctive qualifications which can be entered in its own registers.

The analogies in the processes of controlling undergraduate medical education in the nineteenth century and in professions related to medicine are too obvious to require emphasis. They are all responses, formally organized, to cope with specialization and the complexity of relationships within medicine and within the society that it serves. Each new organization is like a biological species struggling to establish its own life within its environment, both professional and lay. Similar processes were to be witnessed in the founding of hospitals, both general and special, in the eighteenth and nineteenth centuries.

About the same time as the rash of new specialist foundations it was realized that the control of undergraduate medical education, for entry to the profession, was no longer enough to meet the needs of medicine and of society. At the turn of the twentieth century it was enough to make the student a duly qualified doctor. He had the knowledge and skills of the period to last him a professional lifetime in the arts and sciences of medicine, surgery and midwifery. The history of specialization and burgeoning knowledge gradually stripped this generality away. The newly qualified doctor was not a complete professional, but only one to be made a professional by further education and training. Of course this was being realized by many doctors already, and few would have dared to undertake, say, surgical operations for which they had not been specially trained, and many underwent, voluntarily, further training after graduating from medical school, and passed higher diploma examinations in order to specialize in a subject of their choice. But in 1953, in the UK, a statutory requirement was introduced that all medical graduates must undertake a year of supervised practical work in hospitals before being admitted fully to the Medical Register. Again this is only a local response which has been echoed in many other parts of the world. It denotes very formally the entry of government into medical education and its control, evincing once again the concern of the public with the quality and standards of its doctors. Still later, in 1979, there was introduced a Vocational Training Act for general practitioners, which exactly prescribes the experience that they must have before being admitted to government lists as independent practitioners.

A further response within medicine for coping with specialization and the ever-increasing knowledge and skills required for practice has come with formalization of educational programmes for those who have graduated and become registered medically. No doctor now can rest on his laurels after passing his undergraduate examinations and obtaining a degree. He has to enter a graduate programme leading to some further qualification attesting to his specialization. This even applies to general practice, general medicine and general surgery, which despite their persisting names are specialties. No one can cover and practise in the whole of these subjects. Specialties within them have split off and have left an ever-diminishing core, which has therefore taken on aspects of a specialty. To cope with this further education of graduates in medicine, whether junior or senior, organizations have had to be built up in all advanced countries. They vary somewhat from place to place though they all move along the old educational lines requiring prescribed experience for certain lengths of time in prescribed places under supervision and the work done is assessed and examined, at least in the earlier stages of progression. Even for the more senior the same general system is creeping in occasionally.

Educational bodies such as the Royal Colleges and their Faculties have taken over the function of setting standards to be attained for specialization, and in countries other than the UK different agencies have been pressed into service. In the UK the whole National Health Service has been used locally, under the aegis of universities, to provide further education for doctors. The system was set up after the remarkable Christ Church Conference at Oxford in 1961. This brought together Colleges, government, universities, educationalists and many others to formalize the pattern. Again details are unimportant for the moment, but the new pattern demonstrates once more the interactions both within the medical profession and its various bodies and with those of society.

The control of medicine in the interests of society has proceeded even further and apace in the second half of the twentieth century. The war of 1939–45, in Britain, had brought an intensity of effort into all aspects of national life, which had its effects in medicine. There were scientific advances in physics, chemistry, engineering, materials and technology which began to rub off into medicine. These emerged into blood transfusion, anaesthesia, pharmacology, prosthetics, chemotherapy and antibiotics, as well as into radiology and imaging of all types. There were social adjustments too. Army, navy and air force personnel had their own free health and medical advice as a necessary part of waging war. The civilian health services were pressed into service since the UK was a total military base from which operations of war had to be conducted. This put the civilian population at risk, especially from air raids. Great efforts had to be put into the evacuation of people, the hospitals and the health care services, away from the major cities which might be the objects of aerial bombardment. But above all there was a sense of togetherness of the people and a concern for each other's welfare, generating a national feeling of goodwill towards all others.

The coming together of all these various strands emerged in the National Health Act of 1946, under the aegis of Aneurin Bevan, who was then Minister of Health in the government. He rose to his famous achievement of founding the British National Health Service on this wave of social concern and scientific advance. His was by no means a lone voice. There was especially Lord Beveridge with his earlier Report on social insurance and health, and in a different sphere R.A. Butler with an Education Act of 1944. All exemplified the general movement for building a new and better society out of the ashes of the old, burned by the fires of war. Moreover, for health the time was especially ripe. The expensive hospitals, formerly dependent on charity, had been brought under the umbrella of the Ministry of Health, for they needed to be organized to deal with all the vicissitudes of war, and none but government could do this. At the end of the war, when everyone had become used to government and its funds paying for almost everything, there was not enough money from charitable sources to fund the hospitals. In the intervening years they had become even more expensive to run. Their standards were improved and science and technology had given them more efficacious things to do, but all at greatly increased cost. It was inevitable that in some shape or another the government would have to step in. The climate of opinion and conditions of the time demanded it.

The result was the National Health Service which began in 1948 (*Figure 11.1*). It has of course evolved and changed since that day, but essentially it meant that all hospitals and their staffs were taken over and run by government agencies; that general practitioners remained as independent contractors, paid a capitation fee for each patient nominally on their lists; and that public health services remained with

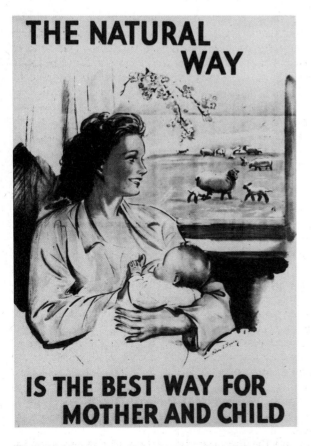

Figure 11.1 British poster issued in 1948. (Reproduced by courtesy of the Wellcome Institute Library, London)

the local government authorities. Later reorganizations have pulled the public health services into the general NHS services, but left those of the general practitioners much as they were. Again for present purposes the details are not important. The trends, though, are. They are similar, *mutatis mutandis*, in many other parts of the world.

For centuries, even millennia, the transactions between doctors and their individual patients as well as their societies have seemed relatively simple and easily understood. There was the doctor and his patient in consultation. Yet always hovering shadowy in the background was the ethos of the profession, its professional conscience, as it were, pervaded by some form of education. This was known to Hippocrates in his Oath with its emphasis on right behaviour by doctors towards their patients and students. So even since antiquity the simple consultation had a third party in it in the presence of ethics hazily understood by doctor and patient and never formally stated. There was another strand too in public health. Here as we have seen the doctors co-operated with authorities to get non-specific measures of hygiene, sanitation, housing, education, pure food and water supplies accepted, so that individuals might be shielded from some of the worst that flesh is heir to. In the armed forces medical and health services these moves for the public and for individuals are more obvious.

Both prevention and cure have to be practised to maintain the fitness of the troops for their fighting and support tasks. There has always too been the problem of who pays the doctor. In the simpler paradigm this was obviously the patient himself (or relatives or other personal supporters). The ability to pay automatically rations access to medical attention. Those who cannot afford it have to do without, unless they can find a third party to pay. Often this was through charity provided by cities, churches, monasteries and religious and lay foundations. Doctors themselves often contributed by giving some of their services free. Yet however good this system was in parts and for its times, it could never reach all those with medical and health needs.

The only alternative to private funds or charity that has been devised is that of insurance. In this, large numbers make some contribution in the hope that only few will actually need to have money spent on them. There have been myriad local schemes of this nature—medical clubs or co-operatives. In the UK they have become especially remembered in connection with mining communities, where the miners and sometimes mine owners made regular contributions so that a doctor could be employed to care for the men and their wives and children. These self-help groups were widened with the National Insurance Act of 1911, whose provisions allowed for some delivery of medical care to those and their families who had to contribute. This was the famous 'panel', and many doctors drew their incomes from treating these patients in return for a salary or capitation fee. The scheme did not cover everybody nor the whole range of available medical care and technology. That icing on the basic cake still came essentially from charity and to some extent from government funds for a few hospitals and dispensaries. Nevertheless, the general themes can be seen developing towards the ideal of medical care for all, whoever they are and wherever they are in the country concerned. This came to fruition imperfectly in the start of the National Health Service in the UK in 1948. This is financed, however it may be disguised, partly by insurance and partly by government funds raised by taxes.

With the rise of specialization and the increasingly costly resources needed for the prosecution of modern medical care, using a larger army of health care workers, the insurance principle has had to spread, at least in the western world. Sometimes the insurance schemes are privately run and sometimes they are run by government. Whatever system is used the government has controlling supervision of how the funds are used and disbursed. There are obvious gaps too in what insurance funds can pay for, so all governments have to provide subventions for special groups of people such as the old, the pensioners, the young, the mentally sick and handicapped and many others. The point is that however it is looked at there is more often than not a third party who is paying for medical care, and this is no longer purely a transaction between doctor and single patient. The context of medical care has changed because of increased specialization and cost, and the concern of all societies for the welfare of all their members. In one way or another the consultation includes doctor, patient, the medical profession, and society at large, all expressing themselves through a variety of formal and informal organizations. Ultimately those who pay, whether government or private insurance agencies, want to know just what it is they are paying for. They then want to know in greater detail what is going on in each consultation, what advice is being given and why, what resources are being employed to carry out treatment, and how much it will all cost.

In other words those who provide the finance are not content just with being told by the doctors that they are using the money and resources properly; the providers want hard evidence that that is just what the medical profession is doing. So it is that in the USA there arose the Professional Standards Review Organization (PSRO). Other countries are following suit, within their own cultural and political contexts.

It is not proposed to pursue the matter further here, but simply to note that out of specialization, high technology and increasing cost of medical care have arisen incursions by organs of society into medical care with incessant frequency. In the historical pattern sketched here it became inevitable, and will continue. A partial defence put up by medicine to the inroads of society into its affairs has been the establishment of medical insurance to protect the doctor if he should be subjected to proceedings for malpractice. This too is a response in the dialogue between medicine and society, occasioned by heightened awareness of each by the other. Adding to the concerns of society with medicine have been many groups devoted to special issues such as poliomyelitis, multiple sclerosis, mental handicap, old age, improving maternity services, patients in general and their care, diabetes, congenital abnormalities and many, many more. They are often self-help clubs in the first instance but then widen their interest to aid research into subjects close to their hearts and through this and other means they form pressure groups to try to influence political and medical processes.

This has had to be a brief sketch of the relationships of medicine as a whole with society as a whole and also of the relationships of parts of medicine and parts of society. The interactions are increasing and daily become more complex. Some social insights and theories are essential to be able to make some sense of what is happening and how. The ramifications of medicine and of health care extend so far that simple paradigms are not enough for comprehension. Yet all too often doctors themselves, as well as politicians, economists, financiers, and patient pressure groups take too simple a view in deciding on what they believe their right actions should be. This is done on the basis of credulous restricted notions about the nature of medicine and its place in society, over-emphasizing the simplicity of direct patient–doctor contacts. This is where medicine is most obviously manifest, but it is immensely more than this now. The substructure on which this too easy concept rests requires social, political, ethical and medical insights derived from history. Such consideration is still too rarely given to medicine. If it were there would be some chance that blinkers might be thrown off and wider and different perspectives given. There might even come more patience and tolerance in the dealings between medicine and society.

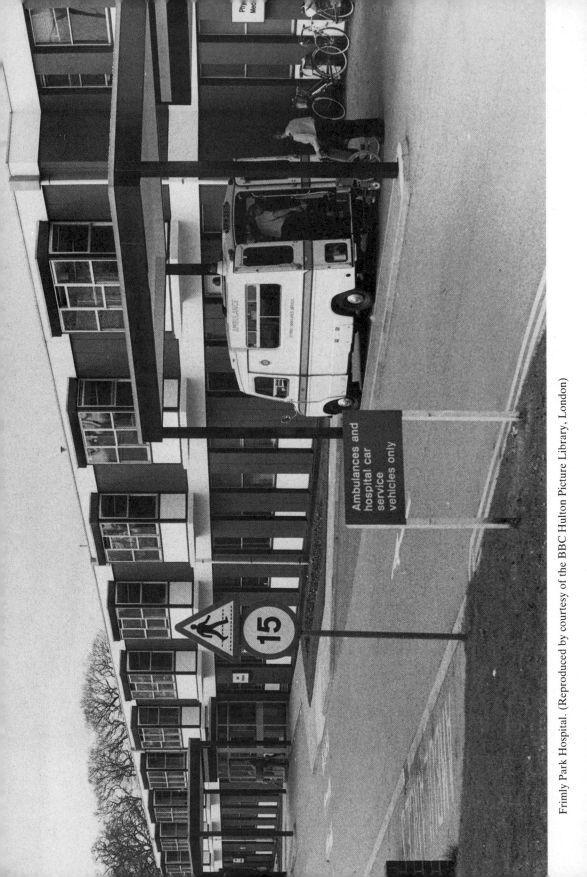

Frimly Park Hospital. (Reproduced by courtesy of the BBC Hulton Picture Library, London)

Chapter 12

Philosophies of medicine

The background thinking that imbues the practice of medicine has varied in different times and places. Such thoughts are presuppositions, preconceptions and assumptions, which are often unexpressed. Yet it is these that are important for determining the directions in which medicine will be allowed to move, both scientifically and socially. It is as though there were a continually varying, scarcely audible hum pervading the air, from which a few gifted people are able to abstract a few notes and sometimes snatches of a tune. The term philosophy is used in this sense, as depicting a form of enquiry into those normally unobserved things that contribute to what is believed to be medical progress. Formal histories of medicine tend to pick out the names of the erudite and the discoveries and advances they have made. Here the intention is to try to discern something of the groundswell on which they have raised themselves to peaks of achievement.

The enduring factors in medicine have always been compassion, pity, care and love. These make nursing the really fundamental aspect of health care. Before there was any formal organization of medicine, however simple and crude, the care of the sick fell on family and friends, and especially on women—the specialists in tenderness, nurture and comfort of all around them, but especially of those who are ill. It is astonishing to contemplate how this somewhat vague general idea has worked itself out over the centuries into the complexities of health care which have formed something of the subject matter of previous chapters. This essential substrate of compassion should never be forgotten in considering the driving forces in the advance of medicine in all its aspects and specializations. Of course that central theme may be interpreted through the years in many different ways. Sometimes it will seem to be entirely submerged in wrangling. Sometimes it is just assumed to be present when it is not. But in total progress it is always there in some form or another. There are daily reminders both within and outside medicine that the needs of patients, people and clients must not be forgotten, especially in an age of science and technology, when it may appear that humane values could be lost.

Even in the most primitive societies there are those, both men and women, who specialize to some extent in the care of the sick and seem to the non-professional to have unusual knowledge of disease and its causes. Such early specialists often unconsciously deceive not only their patients but themselves, believing that they know and understand more than in fact they do. This may be especially so when they call on supernatural powers and try to control them through magic and religion. That they do use these two is some evidence of an underlying philosophy of the time. There is great variety in religion, belief and magic and the practitioners of them all have their own interpretations of disease and their own remedies. This really is private medicine as distinct from public, useable medical knowledge. There can be no common ground between practitioners of any kind until communication and agreement on definitions, aims and objectives is established among them, even if only implicitly. When this happens a corpus of public knowledge, restricted to perhaps a few, begins. It can be taught to others who can also use it. Communication, information and education are the life-blood of any society. They need not be accurate or true by modern standards, but if they are acknowledged and accepted generally then the society can function within its conventions. As mentioned earlier, magic and religion are still parts of medicine. They may not be parts of the scientific corpus of medicine, but they are in the hearts of many patients and are often invoked by them. Doctors may even practise forms of magic by suggestion and they may carry a religious aura even when they may profess no religion. Beliefs in the supernatural are not expunged simply because science does not want them within its fold.

By the time of classical Egyptian and Greek antiquity there were the beginnings of a recognizable medical profession, which was not sharply delineated from others. There came some rational clinical observation together with classification of diseases and their causes. These were very imperfect because the background philosophy was inadequate to explain and interpret phenomena. The beliefs of the time did not allow for a dispassionate consideration of the facts of observation. It is certain though that no fact stands in isolation. It is always related to other facts, but even more importantly it is overlaid with interpretation derived from the climate of opinion of its time and place. Every branch of scientific medicine develops its own climate which blinkers vision as well as directs it. It prevents the consideration of ideas and facts outside its confines.

The early development of the profession brought with it the duties to be expected of a doctor. These are well set out in the Hippocratic Oath. Consideration for others is its keynote, and this stemmed from the philosophy of the time with some emphasis on the equal importance of each individual. This was a philosophical ideal rather than reality, for many of the Greek city-states were based in slavery. Nevertheless the idea was important subsequently for the whole western world in fostering democracy and for the developments of medicine in it. The medical power for influencing the lives of others has to be used carefully and with due ethical concern. Certain things may be done, but not others, and the confidences of all patients must be respected and preserved. It is in this that trust between doctor and patient is established and preserved. It is so old a concept that it is automatically expected by all in western civilization, however often there are attempts for many reasons to breach it.

This trust between the professions and the individuals whom they serve is a bastion of freedom against the encroachments of society as exemplified in government and many of its agencies as well as in other people singly or in informal groups. The struggle between private confidences and the right of the public to know—about the activities and behaviour of those who constitute it—in order to judge whether society's rights are being infringed will ever continue. The professions, including that of medicine, are at one end of the spectrum protecting individuality, while government, law, police, media and the revenue are at the other. The general statement about confidentiality is easy to subscribe to. In difficult instances where private and public duties conflict there has to be specific testing of the rights and wrongs by legal process or professional judgement. The consideration for others in the Oath is a further extension of the general duty of compassion mentioned previously.

The Greek views of the world were founded in introspection, contemplation and speculation, with very little basis in organized natural observation. Inevitably, therefore, there could be no great scientific advances in the present tradition. The world view of the time did not allow development then in that direction. The Greek beliefs held sway for centuries. Transmuted though they are, they still do. Their impact is incalculable and rivalled only by that of Christianity. In essence these two exemplify the rational, scientific and the emotional needs of western Man. (This is not to suggest that science is always rational, nor that religion is always emotional.) Christianity gave religious force to the importance of the individual and also reinforced concern and consideration for mankind, since all are equal in the sight of God. There have been many aberrations in the application of these basic important ideas throughout history, but the general tenor of compassion, mercy and love reinforced by belief in them as divinely inspired have been and remain of benefit to medicine. Religion has made them more formal and more of a duty, almost a form of worship. One of the unforeseen sideshoots of Christian development was that sciences, arts, education and civil affairs were mainly taken into the hands of the clergy. We have seen how, with thoughts centred on God and the life to come, science and medicine tended to be in limbo. If this life is a vale of tears with much better to come after death the struggle for more life through the intervention of medicine seems vain. This attitude stifled enquiry, and especially into the prime basic science of medicine, anatomy. The body was the vehicle for the soul and therefore ought not ever to be defiled and especially after death.

Medical scientific endeavour in Christian Roman times and in the Middle Ages was not entirely stopped, as we have seen. There were still some insights, mainly in surgery, since this is essentially simple in concept. Moreover, the Roman legions marched all over Europe and needed medical support, both in tending soldiers' injuries and in keeping the troops healthy by environmental and public health measures, especially in sanitation, warmth, clothing and food supply. Similar measures went ahead in the cities subjected to Roman influence. These environmental controls may not then have been recognized as medical, but they did contribute to the health or otherwise of populations. Their relevance to medicine has become apparent only over later centuries. The concept of what medicine is, and what its concerns are, have widened beyond the simplistic notion that it is a matter of a single doctor in contact with a single patient. That concept still lingers on and distorts assumptions about the range of modern medicine. The doctor–patient relationship is central, but more and more factors now impinge on it and modify it.

With the Renaissance, new trains of thought in many spheres were ushered in, but especially in science. This can now be seen to be comparable with Greek philosophy and the Christian religion in its importance for western civilization. The first phase was that of observation of nature, with a little experiment. In this movement there is no need to reiterate what has gone before. Gradually experiment has become triumphant. Instead of simply observing nature, it has been put to the test. But observation and experiment alone have no significance unless and until they are related to a theoretical background, a philosophy, which binds the observations and experiments together into a more coherent whole. This is the

importance of Newton, Darwin, Einstein and others, for they introduced a
generality of coherence into what had previously been disparate and discrete. They
made sense of at least parts of the world of nature. Facts, so-called, are invested
with a penumbra of interpretation which is concordant with accepted beliefs. These
form a common culture developed by communication in its infinite variety. This
community is made more comprehensible by psychological and sociological theory,
which are products of the twentieth century. They became possible when some of
the physical vicissitudes of life were made more bearable. Until there is food,
clothing, warmth, shelter and productive leisure in relative abundance there is little
room for theorizing. But when the physical needs are largely met then mental and
social phenomena can have a greater place in the intellectual scheme of things.

Now it remains to be seen where the old driving forces of society and of medicine
have led, and to attempt to discern what is in the background of present medical
thought and practice. The old ideals are still there though they have been modified
and stressed in different ways. Above all it would seem that it is science that has
taken hold, together with the technology based on it. The results of this have
surpassed the wildest prevision. Nothing seems beyond the reach of scientific
enquiry properly conducted and given time. And yet that is how their systems
seemed to Greek philosophers and Christian theologians. Each of them took in and
explained everything of significance and importance. To the modern all-embracing
scientist, however, these two 'systems' are irrelevant and have been passed by.
(There are, of course, no such extreme scientists quite as unaware of other worlds
about them than those of science; nor, one might presume, were there such totally
extreme philosophers and theologians. But constant qualification of general
statements has to stop somewhere.) The fact that all systems of thought and
virtually all civilizations are superseded should give science some pause before
arrogating too much and becoming an insatiate cormorant.

The triumphs of modern medicine and biology have been in cellular biology. The
atomism of the physical atoms was broken down, and so was that of the cell. More
and more particles and little systems are discovered within the supposed integrated
units. There is a dependence of everything on everything else. The organelles are
built up into cells, the cells into organs, the organs into systems, the systems into
individuals and the individuals into societies. The whole is made up of parts, and
the parts, when integrated, produce something that would not have been foreseen.
A traveller from outer space given some organelles or cells or even a heap of organs
would probably not be able to forecast how they might ultimately come together to
give rise to Man, with mental powers and the ability to form societies. It may be of
importance that the 'lower levels' of corporeal existence give insight into the
'higher levels', but one has to be aware of those higher levels before gaining the
insights. The lower levels have to be visualized in relationship with a whole. The
whole could not be predicted purely from the parts. The smaller those parts the less
their predictive value becomes. Knowledge of a metabolic chain makes no sense in
isolation. The method of science is therefore in medicine one of anatomizing, that
is of 'cutting up' into smaller and smaller parts. I.A. Richards put it neatly in saying
that 'scientific method (is) the method of considering, whenever possible, one thing
at a time'. This allows some experimental control of what is being investigated. The
field of indeterminacy is then decreased and changes within a smaller system can be
understood when those within a very large system cannot, because too much is
being presented for attention at any one time, and the parts cannot be controlled
and held steady.

This matter of being unable to predicate the whole individual from a knowledge of its smaller parts is reinforced by consideration of what seems to happen with sudden death, as for instance in a car crash, or when an insect may be crushed underfoot. All the atoms and molecules of the creature are still present in the immediate vicinity. In this restricted sense nothing has been lost, though an immense change has been wrought. It is obvious when somebody is alive one minute and is dead the next. 'Life' has gone out of the corpse, or the 'soul' has departed were the old descriptions. In a scientific sense what has gone is the organization and integration of millions, even billions, of smaller systems. Life seems to be integration piled on integration. Integration is impermanent while only the subatomic particles are eternal. That is now the world view that modern science seems to accept. The individual is a temporary organizer of physical matter within his envelope. When he dies there is slow disintegration of the material which is returned to a general pool, so that its atoms and molecules can be taken up into other systems.

Every aspect of nature—seas, shores, mountains, fields, hedges, forests, deserts, cities, societies, everything—is a shifting, changing kaleidoscope of systems in varying relationships with one another. All at base are combinations of subatomic particles, which seem to be the only more or less permanent things, and even they are capable of many metamorphoses. There is a certain permanence in an oxygen atom (say) trapped in a molecule deep inside a mountain, but even it is moving and may be changing its relationships with other atoms and molecules close by. In the course of 'infinite' time it may move to the surface, be washed away by rain or be blown off by the wind, end up in a river, be ingested by a fish, which is eaten by a man, who for a time incorporates it in his tissues, from which the oxygen atom may be released by metabolic process, or be returned to the general pool after death by bacterial and enzymatic action or by cremation. The whole concept is breathtaking in its sweep and comprehensiveness. The immanence of change and process, the building up and the breaking down, the use of comparatively few simple particles to fashion the whole of the observed world rearranged and joined together should leave us 'lost in wonder, love and praise'. The basic materials are a seething, writhing mass out of which some sort of order that we can observe emerges.

As regards the origin of life it seems that simpler molecules combine, draw envelopes round themselves, begin some control of their immediate (intracellular) environment, keeping the 'extracellular' environment at bay, yet drawing on it for metabolism and excretion, then making complex molecules as templates on which the original system may be replicated. It is the process of reproduction—in which temporary integrations, by design, are repeatedly brought into being—that to our minds distinguishes living from non-living processes. This is the message of genetics so that offspring are recognizably a likeness of their parents. Yet offspring do vary slightly from their parents, even when they are cells produced by binary fission. They do things slightly differently from their forebears. This alters relationships both within and outside them. This is the basis of biological evolution, making all the old materials combine and recombine in ever-increasing ways. Life of a kind is everywhere, invading and exploiting the resources provided by the physical world, yet returning its materials to it after using them for shorter or longer periods.

The evolutionary process is described as moving from cells to multicellular organisms, then on to differentiation and growth, through to tissues, organs and systems in never-ending succession. Out of the simple inorganic arises the organic leading ultimately to Man. The driving force is unknown. There is no answer within science to the question of why it all happens. The why is left to religions. Science supplies answers only to how. But the triumphs of science do have their effects on religions. Both science and religion try to give a total world view, with religion claiming a greater power to interpret the meaning of the universe. The result is that science appears always to be encroaching on what once were religious preserves. Then religions seem to be in retreat. This is a very definite factor in the changes in thinking of western societies, and it has been much emphasized previously how dependent science and medicine are on the cultural views held in the societies of which they are a part.

The scientific and medical philosophy just sketched leaves no room for life after death, and so cuts deeply into the foundations of many religions. At death the individual in a corporeal sense disappears for ever. His influence may live on, much transmuted, in those who have been affected by it. Just as his physical substance slowly disintegrates and is scattered widely, with less and less recognition of his individuality, so does his intellectual influence become diluted after his death. This raises a philosophical dilemma for medicine which has still scarcely been realized. It begs the question of what is medicine for? What is its purpose? It satisfies a deep-felt need as this history shows, but why? The question is unanswerable in that form. It was answerable, and for some still is, in religious terms, but these are no longer universally acceptable. The extent of this opposition to religious tenets may perhaps be seen in the legalizing of abortions and the increased rate of performing them, in doubts about prolonging the lives of the economically unproductive old, chronic sick and mentally and physically handicapped, and so in euthanasia. There is still a belief in the importance of each individual based in Greek philosophy and Christianity (and other religions) but in the idiom of science the question has been changed so that it has become 'to what extent is each life important?' It is the nature of science always to wish to measure and quantify, to see things simply and unequivocally, preferably in mathematical symbols.

Although death may be explicable in scientific terms as disintegration, there is more difficulty with the evolution of mind. Philosophically Descartes separated mind from body in the seventeenth century. The idea persists in most thinking, even within medicine. Yet there is no scientific evidence of mind after death of the brain; various mental states can be induced by drugs acting chemically on the brain; disordered mental states can be improved in similar fashion by drugs or by physical and surgical means. In short, there is no mind without body and body is a complex interweaving of chemical systems. Things are no better when the evolutionary series of animals is contemplated. Many of them show what must be called mental activity. And in genetic material some have affected to see a form of memory. The DNA remembers what it must do to perpetuate the species and then it programs the chemical materials at hand to make them produce a replicated individual of the species. There is much more evidence to be adduced to show that the old dualism of mind and body is no longer adequate as a philosophical basis for the long-standing problems of their interrelationships. Yet medicine simply takes no notice, preferring to see some phenomena as mental and some as physical, and most diseases as a combination of the two. It remains pragmatic and not apparently worried by inconsistencies.

Psychiatry itself is among the most ambivalent of subjects. Colloquially the practitioners have been designated as either 'druggers' or 'talkers'. They use different philosophical bases, believing in either the chemistry of mind explaining everything or in the separateness (or near separateness) of mind and body. Yet somewhere chemical processes become mental and some mental ones become chemical, as when there is a will to move a limb or to talk. This same problem besets theologians too. For them there is the matter of free will, and therefore that of predestination and the individual's power to sin and to repent. The chemical view of mind seems to lead directly to determinism in which every action, every thought would appear to be dictated by the chemical reactions immediately preceding the overt behaviour.

This takes too simple a view of the complexity and potential variability of chemical responses that are possible at the brain's high level of integration. It is worth consideration that it may be artificial to try to separate brain from mind. It may be that they are simply aspects of the same thing and that it is our preconceptions and categorization that make for the difficulties of reconciliation of the two apparently distinct things. In the course of history we have seen how the boundaries between energy and matter, between physics and chemistry, between chemistry and biology, betweeen living and non-living, between living and mental phenomena have become blurred and have disappeared. There is only continuity and no discontinuity, except that which is put there by ourselves in order to reduce an overwhelming plethora of fact and information to some system. In other words it may be ourselves who put the divisions into nature, rather than the divisions being real. By analogy therefore it could be that it is we who separate mind from body and make it too big a problem. For our own purposes we need to distinguish them, but they could be simply aspects of the same thing, with us feeling that we want a different frame of reference for each aspect.

It may seem that considerations of the great themes of life and death, of matter and mind, of living and non-living, have comparatively little to do with the history of medicine. Yet a moment's thought will show that it is these themes that underlie and determine much of the nature of medical practice. They are therefore highly relevant to questions posed by the care of the dying, the extent of surgery and of other treatments for cancer, the proper care of the mentally ill, the mentally and physically handicapped and the chronic sick. They determine the extent to which it is decided that expensive high technologies shall be used in the treatment of the sick, and also when life-support machines shall be turned off or maintain a person in a semblance of life.

The arguments for and against various policies to be pursued in all these debatable areas rarely note that at bottom they rest in assumptions about the value of life and in attitudes to death, to illness and to handicap. The arguments proceed from premises in philosophy, religion and science which are not stated, as they ought to be. The arguments are derivative, yet what they are derived from is not stated. There is no wonder that agreements on policies cannot be reached. The contestants have no common intellectual ground and do not even recognize the fact. Since ethical problems are probably the most important for medicine at the present time it would be sensible to formulate philosophies more precisely than has so far been the case.

These fundamental attitudes to medicine are determined in some degree by the political milieux in which it is practised. A political system too is one expression of an underlying philosophy or approach to life. The medical practice in a dictatorship is different from that in a thoroughgoing democracy. It is not intended to consider further these matters of politics and philosophy. It is enough that it should be realized that medicine is dependent upon them and in various ways is both constrained and liberated by them, but it cannot be practised as if they did not exist. This is one of the major lessons that the medical profession is having to learn in the later twentieth century.

The major philosophical stance of medicine and the attitudes to it consciously expressed or unexpressed by the medical profession now are those of science. It has already been suggested that this, when completely adopted, leads to some discarding and much modification of Greek philosophical and Christian with other religious traditions. The fact needs recognition and some decision. It should not be simply ignored, as in general it is. All the strands in the development of medicine need some formal appraisal in the light of history, to try to make sure that the threads that continue to be valuable are not jettisoned, and that those that no longer have use are abandoned. The question must be whether a totally scientific approach to medicine is a satisfactory one. For the present the answer must be a resounding 'no'.

There are still too many areas of life and of medicine that are inexplicable in scientific terms. Other frames of reference then have to be used—humanitarian, ethical, cultural, religious and other. The world and its phenomena have to be carved up by the human mind in different ways to try to make sense of them. No one method of carving explains everything so far. The preconceptions behind each method are valid for the particular method but may be intellectually irreconcilable with others.

For medicine and biology the broad scientific proceeding has been to take the body and anatomize it into organs and systems, then to cells and tissues and later to biochemical, chemical, and physical mechanisms, giving explanations of phenomena at all these levels. Only with the twentieth century have there been moves to the other levels of psychology and sociology. The lower levels (the ones dealing with ever smaller parts) do not always fully explain the behaviour of the higher ones. Indeed, random behaviour with increased complexity of response seems to be one of the essentials of biological and human evolution. In the isolation of laboratory conditions a very small process will develop in only one way (within limits). But if that defined process is put in association and relationships with others, the outcome is unpredictable in simple terms. The organization of simple process with simple process brings out something other than might have been foreseen. A pile of bricks does not indicate what the form of the ultimate building will be. It is the incredible assembling, assorting and re-assorting of basic materials in biology that is a cause for wonder. The same building bricks are used repeatedly in different combinations to produce the variety of the living world, from viruses and bacteria, through tiny plants and animals and up to trees and Man. Similar basic plans are discernible in all of them. The raw materials are comparatively few.

In moving from lower to higher levels of consideration certainty seems to get less and less. This is only partially true, for physicists, who seem to gain the most certainty from their investigations, also find much uncertainty. Their particles often do not behave as might be expected from previous experience with them. Though matter at these levels appears to be constrained by physical and mathematical laws which ought to predict behaviour accurately, it is often found that some of it behaves randomly. This may be very important philosophically, for as the scale of levels is ascended there seems to be an increase in the potentiality for variations in behaviour. Apparently identical people subjected to the same stimulus may behave quite differently. The results of such interactions are only predictable statistically, which means that of a large group many will behave in one way and some in a variety of different ways. It is the randomness that is quantifiable, though the performance of one individual will remain unpredictable.

It may be this that right from the beginning predicated mind and intelligence, and it may again show that body and mind are simply different aspects of the same thing—different ways of the human mind for carving up the phenomena of the world for contemplation and investigation. These different ways demand different techniques, as the specializations in medicine, the sciences, the arts and religions demonstrate. History shows that there is no mandate for any one approach to take over from all the others. It is arrogant for any one of them to assume that it has the only worth-while approach to the truth. It is in the nature of the newest in human affairs to try to dominate and take over. Science is the relative newcomer at present. The others were novel in previous centuries.

The philosophical problem of the late twentieth century in medicine is the assumption that science, with the technology it spawns and derives from, will provide the answers to illness and the preservation of health. The success of the scientific approach has been so great in the past hundred years that it would be surprising if that assumption were not made. In an historical perspective the belief would seem to be unrealistic. Science will continue to have its triumphs but they will not be and cannot be all-conquering. The opposition to this naïve idea is already building up. 'There are more things in heaven and earth, Horatio, than are dreamt of in your philosophy.'

Education is conventionally divided up into knowledge, skills and attitudes. Knowledge and skills are the provinces of science and technology. As we have seen these proceed apace in medicine. There is no stopping them, even if that were desirable. The momentum is such within medicine that they will continue to flourish and can be left to take care of themselves, as they undoubtedly will. It is attitudes both inside and outside medicine, however, that should be the present concern. It is they that determine how, when and where knowledge and skills should be and will be exercised. These two give evidence about what can be done, but not whether and how much they should do. This is why philosophy, in the sense used here, is so important to medicine. Ideas and especially systems of ideas are the substrate on which actions are based, even though there are dialogues between ideas and actions. Actions do not just arise. They have a background in thought. This can be inexplicit and later obscured by the results of action.

The next move in medicine, already begun, will probably be to make a more formal consideration of attitudes to it and within it. History and philosophy are necessary ingredients in the understanding and direction of medicine in the future, so that it might continue to serve society and remain in valuable relationships with it, remembering the multitude of societies that have come and gone and the medical systems that have formed part of them. The reactions between them have continually changed and will go on doing so. An understanding of this, derived partly from history, is liberating and leads to tolerance of the aberrations in general progress.

Select bibliography

To those who have read this book it should be obvious that the history of medicine is not to be considered in isolation from general history, nor of the history of science, literature and philosophy. Many excellent general histories can be found on the paperback bookshelves. The same is true of the histories of special subjects. The benefit of being an amateur is the freedom to be catholic in taste and inclination, whereas the professional must bury himself in detail. Biographies of famous doctors number thousands and may be obtained through libraries, though quick reference to life histories can always be made through the *Encyclopaedia Britannica* and other works such as the forthcoming *Oxford Companion to Medicine,* to be published in 1985.

The following list includes the books that I have found of most use in writing this work. I have drawn freely on their ideas, culled over many years of reading, and on their details in the drafting of the manuscript. For these I am especially grateful for the books by Guthrie, Garrison, Singer and Morton. I owe them all an immense debt for the pleasure they have given me in the past and for guiding my footsteps during recent months as I wrote. Without them I could not even have started.

BERNAL, J.D. (1965). *Science in History,* 3rd edn (4 Volumes). Harmondsworth: Penguin Books. Very interesting in detail and in background, though with political overtones of Communism. Volume 3 is the most useful and is called *The Natural Sciences in Our Time*

COBBAN, A. (ed.) (1969) *The Eighteenth Century*. London: Thames and Hudson. A general work but gives a flavour of the time and also its thinking

CORSI, P. and WEINDLING, P. (eds) (1983). *Information Sources in the History of Science and Medicine.* London: Butterworths. An indispensable guide. A series of essays on many aspects of the subject, each followed with references to key publications

DUBOS, R. (1960). *Mirage of Health*. London: George Allen and Unwin. Subtitled *Utopias, Progress and Biological Change.* Effective exposition of the certainty that there is no health that will be lasting and unchanging. Life is struggle and there is no static permanence to be had in a dynamic world

DUNCAN, A.S., DUNSTAN, G.R. and WELBOURN, R.B. (eds) (1981). *Dictionary of Medical Ethics*, Revised ed. London: Darton, Longman and Todd. A series of short articles designed to give a start with a perceived problem in medical ethics. Very good. Browsing through it will awaken many questions previously never even thought of

EISELEY, L. (1958). *The Immense Journey*. London: Victor Gollancz. (1959). *Darwin's Century (Evolution and the Men who Discovered it)*. London: Victor Gollancz. (1961). *The Firmament of Time.* London: Victor Gollancz. A vastly entertaining writer about evolution. *Darwin's Century* is especially noteworthy for its tracing of the history of ideas about evolution

Encyclopaedia Britannica. (1975). 15th edn. Chicago. Indispensable. Excellent articles for the general reader. Many potted biographies of the famous for easy reference

FRASER, J.T. (ed.) (1968). In *The Voices of Time,* London: The Penguin Press. A series of articles on the notion of time as seen from the point of view of different philosophies, by horologists, physicists and biologists and others

GARRISON, F.H. (1929). *An Introduction to the History of Medicine,* 4th edn. Philadelphia: W.B. Saunders Company. A big book, invaluable as a source of reference. Seems to concentrate on published works and on brief biographies. Difficult to discern general movements of thought, which are lost in important detail. Fine to fill in the broad framework when that is known

GLOYNE, S.R. (1950). *John Hunter.* Edinburgh: Livingstone

GRAHAM, H. (1950). *Eternal Eve.* London: Heinemann. The best comprehensive account of the history of obstetrics and gynaecology. An example of a bad title

GUTHRIE, D. (1945). *A History of Medicine.* London: Thomas Nelson and Sons. This is one of the best short histories. Naturally enough, it has nothing to say of the past 50 years. A most excellent general introduction

HAGGARD. H.W. *Devils, Drugs and Doctors.* London: Heinemann. (No date of publication). Good in parts, in outlining medical history

JANSSENS, P.A. (1970). *Palaeopathology (Diseases and Injuries of Prehistoric Man).* London: John Baker

KLEIN, R. (1983). *The Politics of the National Health Service.* London: Longman. A perceptive look at the muddled thinking that was in the background at the start of the NHS, and that still remains. There has never been a well-thought-out and consistent philosophy about what the NHS is for and how it should pursue its course. This book teases out some of the conflicting policies that continue to plague the NHS

LLOYD, G.E.R. (ed.) (1978). *Hippocratic Writings.* London: Penguin Books

MEDAWAR, P.B. (1975). *The Uniqueness of the Individual.* London: Methuen. (1960). *The Future of Man.* London: Methuen. (1967). *The Art of the Soluble.* London: Methuen. (1969). *Induction and Intuition in Scientific Thought.* London: Methuen. (1977). *The Life Science* (with MEDAWAR, J.S.). London: Wildwood House. A series of books by one of Britain's most distinguished biologists, with a direct interest in medicine, especially in immunology. Writes superbly about scientific thinking and philosophy

MORTON, L.T. (1983). *A Medical Bibliography,* 4th edn. Aldershot: Gower Publishing. Its subtitle is *An Annotated Checklist of Texts Illustrating the History of Medicine.* Quite indispensable. Amazing scholarship, with brief notes on the importance of certain publications in the development of each major discipline of medicine. The expert in any one branch can easily recognize significant omissions in his specialty, but this does not diminish the overall value. All students should have access to it

NEWMAN, C. (1957). *The Evolution of Medical Education in the Nineteenth Century.* Oxford University Press. A classic work. Traces its subject through the founding of the General Medical Council and up to the concept that medical education was for the producing of the 'safe general practitioner'—a notion quickly killed by the twentieth century

PATER, J.E. (1981). *The Making of the National Health Service.* London: King Edward's Hospital Fund for London. An insider's view, as a civil servant, of how the NHS came into being, who won the arguments and why

PELLEGRINO, E.D. and THOMASMA, D.C. (1981). *A Philosophical Basis of Medical Practice.* Oxford University Press

PETERSON, J.M. (1978). *The Medical Profession in Mid-Victorian London.* University of California Press. A valuable work showing the dominance of London at this time. Much modern organization of medicine stems from the beliefs and attitudes of physicians and surgeons of the nineteenth century

PHELPS, G. (1979). *A Short History of English Literature.* London: Folio Society

POPPER, K. (1972). *The Logic of Scientific Discovery.* London: Hutchinson. The book which revolutionized thought about the nature of science. Required reading, even though difficult

REEVES, J.W. (1958). *Body and Mind in Western Thought.* Harmondsworth: Penguin Books

REISER, S.J. (1978). *Medicine and the Reign of Technology.* Cambridge University Press. A history of the development of many instruments used in medicine and how they have advanced practice, theory and specialization

RHODES, P. (1976). *The Value of Medicine.* London: George Allen and Unwin

ROBERTS, J.M. (1980). *The Pelican History of the World.* Harmondsworth: Penguin Books. A great ranging over the major happenings in history and the ideas and movements that contributed to them. Essential reading for anyone wishing to be considered generally educated

RUSSELL, B. (1946). *History of Western Philosophy (And its Connections with Political and Social Circumstances from the Earliest Times to the Present Day).* London: George Allen and Unwin. Vital for the amateur

SHOTTER, E.F. (1970). *Matters of Life and Death.* London: Darton, Longman and Todd

SHRYOCK, R.H. (1979). *The Development of Modern Medicine.* University of Wisconsin Press. The subtitle of *An Interpretation of the Social and Scientific Factors Involved* explains something of its purpose. Essential reading, though not intended to be detailed about individuals, any more than the present work

SINGER, C. (1928). *A Short History of Medicine*. Oxford University Press. Another excellent introduction. Traces the history of ideas in medicine very well. The twentieth century is inevitably skimped

TOULMIN, S. and GOODFIELD, J. (1961). *The Fabric of the Heavens*. London: Hutchinson. (1962). *The Architecture of Matter*. London: Hutchinson. (1965). *The Discovery of Time*. London: Hutchinson. A superb trilogy tracing the growth of ideas in astronomy, in physics and about time, and how they have developed in practice

TOYNBEE, A. (1972). *A Study of History*. Oxford University Press and Thames and Hudson. The illustrated edition for the amateur. A real eye-opener. Explores some of the factors leading to the rise and fall of many past civilizations. Read it to stop becoming too arrogant about the future of western civilization, which may not last as long as you thought it might, not because of the 'bomb' or other engines of destruction, but because of inadequate philosophy and values.

WHITEHEAD, A.N. (1943). *Adventures of Ideas*. Cambridge University Press. (1943). *Science and the Modern World*. Cambridge University Press. Still among the best of the philosophers of biology even though he wrote in the 1920s. Amazingly broad sweep of ideas and how they slowly come to fruition over centuries. Sees the essential continuity in all our experiences

WILLEY, B. (1962). *The Seventeenth Century Background*. Harmondsworth: Penguin Books. Explores the thought of the century, mainly through literature, but interesting for scientists and doctors too

ZINSSER, H. (1937). *Rats, Lice and History*. London: George Routledge and Sons. A fascinating account of the natural history and investigation of typhus. Also of human adaptation to syphilis. Outlines how the course of general history may have been modified by epidemics

Chronology

This chronology is brief, incomplete and inexact. Its intention is like that of a route guide—to give a rough sense of direction and some landmarks to look out for, as well as to estimate crudely the time taken between them.

BC

2000	Code of Hammurabi of Babylon
1500	Ebers papyrus
460–370	Hippocrates
450–380	Socrates
429–347	Plato
384–322	Aristotle
338–323	Alexander the Great
310–250	School of Alexandria
c.280	Erasistratus
c.280	Herophilus
c.150	Asclepiades

AD

30	Celsus' *De Re Medicina*
c.130	Soranus of Ephesus
131–201	Galen
150	Ptolemy—astronomer
303	Saints Cosmas and Damian martyred
431	Nestorius banished for heresy
570–632	Mohammed
738	School of Montpellier
860–932	Rhazes
980–1036	Avicenna
1050	Albucasis
1100–80	Salerno's reputation established
1110	University of Paris founded
1126–1198	Averroes
1135–1204	Maimonides
1137	St. Bartholomew's Hospital, London
1158	University of Bologna
1180	University of Montpellier
1201	University of Oxford
1214–1294	Roger Bacon
1215	St. Thomas's Hospital, London

1222	University of Padua
1223	University of Cambridge
1223–1303	Taddeo Alderotti
1227–1274	Thomas Aquinas
1231	Medical School at Salerno established by Frederick II
1300–1368	Guy de Chauliac
1316	Mundinus' *Anathomia*
1330	Gunpowder introduced into warfare
1348–50	Black Death—epidemic bubonic plague
1370	John of Arderne on surgery
1373–5	Boccaccio in Florence
1403	Quarantine in Venice
1440–50	Invention of printing
1452–1519	Leonardo da Vinci
1454	Gutenburg Bible
1473–1543	Copernicus
1474	Caxton's printing press
1478	Celsus' first-century book reprinted
	Mundinus' book reprinted
1479	Avicenna's tenth-century book reprinted
1480	*Regimen Salernitatis*
1486	Latin edition of Rhazes' ninth-century book reprinted
1492	Columbus finds America
	John of Gaddesden
1493–1541	Paracelsus
1494	University of Aberdeen
1496–1500	Syphilis spreads through Europe
1500	Nüfer's caesarean section
1505	Charter of Royal College of Surgeons of Edinburgh
1510–1590	Ambroise Paré
1512–1594	Mercator
1513	Rösslin's *Rosengarten*
1514–1564	Vesalius
1516	More's *Utopia*
1517	Luther at Wittenberg
1517–24	Linacre's translations of Galen (second century)
1518	College of Physicians of London
1519–22	Magellan's voyages round the world
1521–23	Berengario de Carpi on anatomy
1526	Paracelsus on chemical therapy
1530	Fracastoro's *Syphilis sive morbus Gallici*
1536	Paracelsus' *Chirurgia Magna*
1537	Dryander's *Anatomica*
1539	Cardan's theory of probabilities
1540	Guild of Barber–Surgeons
	Raynalde's *The Byrthe of Mankind*
1543	Vesalius' *De Humani Corporis Fabrica*
	Copernicus' *De Revolutionibus Orbum Coelestium*
1546	Fracastoro's *De Contagione*
1549	Cranmer's *Book of Common Prayer*
1550 *et seq.*	Anatomy theatres established in many places
1554	Rueff's book on midwifery
1559	Colombo's *De Re Anatomica*
	Stromayer on ophthalmology
1561	Fallopius' *Observationes Anatomicae*
1564	Eustachius on anatomy
1567	Paracelsus on miner's phthisis
1578	de Baillou on whooping cough
1580	Scurvy on Drake's voyages
1589	Galileo and falling bodies
1590	Jansens introduce compound microscope

1596	Mercurio on midwifery
	Kepler on astronomy
1597	Tagliacozzi on plastic surgery
1600	Gilbert's *De Magnete*
	Bruno burned at stake
	Fabricius *On the Valves of the Veins*
1604	Kepler showed inverted image on retina
1605	Francis Bacon's *Advancement of Learning*
1609	Galileo used telescope
	Sanctorius invented clinical thermometer
	Louise Bourgeois on midwifery
1610	Galileo used microscope
1614	Sanctorius on metabolism
1617	Society of Apothecaries
1620	Pilgrim Fathers in New England
1621	Burton's *Anatomy of Melancholy*
1627	Aselli on lymphatics
1628	Harvey's *De Motu Cordis et Sanguinis*
1632	Galileo establishes Copernican system as against Ptolemaic
1635	Browne's *Religio Medici*
1637	Descartes' *Discours Sur la Methode*
1642	Descartes' *Meditations*
1650	Glisson on rickets
1651	Harvey's *De Generatione Animalium*
1654	Glisson on the liver
1661	Boyle's *The Sceptical Chymist*
	Malpighi demonstrated capillaries
	Descartes on physiology
1662	Graunt analyses bills of mortality
1663	Charter of the Royal Society
1664	Willis on anatomy of the brain
1665	Hooke's *Micrographia*
1667	Hooke on function of the lungs
1668	Mauriceau on midwifery
1670	Clément delivered Marquise de Montespan
1672	de Graaf on ovarian follicles
1677	Bartholin—glands in female perineum
1679	Leeuwenhoek saw spermatozoa
1681	Royal College of Physicians of Edinburgh
1683	Leeuwenhoek saw bacteria
	Petty on vital statistics
1687	Newton's *Principia Mathematica*
1690	Locke's *Essay Concerning Human Understanding*
1693	Halley on vital statistics
1700	Ramazzini on diseases of various trades
1708	Boerhaave's *Institutiones Medicae*
1710	Berkeley's *Essay Towards a New Theory of Vision*
1714	Fahrenheit's thermometer
1719	Westminster Hospital
1721	Guy's Hospital
1726	Gibson in chair of obstetrics in Edinburgh—1st in the world
1732	Boerhaave's *Elementa Chemiae*
1733	Cheselden's *Osteographia*
	Chapman on midwifery first mentions obstetric forceps
	Hales measured blood pressure
1735	Linnaeus' *Systema Naturae*
1736	Shippen teaching obstetrics in USA
1738	Hume's *Treatise on Human Nature*
	Methodism in London
1740	Richardson's *Pamela*
1741	The Foundling Hospital

1742	Celsius' temperature scale
1747	von Haller's *Primae Lineae Physiologica*
1749	Buffon's *Histoire Naturelle*
1752	Smellie's *Treatise on Midwifery*
	Pringle's *Observations on the Diseases of the Army*
1753	Lind's *A Treatise of The Scurvy*
1754	Black finds CO_2; destroys phlogiston theory
1758	Monro II—chair of anatomy at Edinburgh
1759	Wolff's *Theoria Generationis*
1760	Morgagni's *On the Sites and Causes of Disease*
1761	Auenbrugger on percussion
1763	Linnaeus' classification of diseases
1766	Cavendish—CO_2 and H_2
1769	Watt's steam engine
1770	William Hunter's school of anatomy—Windmill Street
1771	Priestley—O_2
1772	Priestley—N_2, N_2O
1774	Hunter's *Anatomy of the Human Gravid Uterus*
1776	Blumenbach classifies human races
1780	Galvani observes twitch of frogs' legs
1782	Spallanzini on digestion
1785	Withering's *An Account of the Foxglove*
1786	John Hunter ligated popliteal aneurysm
1788	Act to protect boys employed by chimney sweeps
1792	Wollstonecraft's *Vindication of the Rights of Women*
	Volta's *Letters on Animal Electricity*
1794	Retreat at York
1795	Gordon on puerperal fever
	Hutton's *Theory of the Earth*
1797	Eden's *The State of the Poor*
1798	Malthus' *Essay on the Principle of Population*
	Jenner on vaccination
	Pinel removed chains from the insane
1800	Royal College of Surgeons (of England)
	Bichat on pathology
1801	First census in Britain
1804	Dalton established Atomic Theory
1806	Davy—Na, K, Mg, Cl
1808	Corvisart on heart and great blood vessels
1809	McDowell's ovariotomy
1811	Avogadro's hypothesis
1812	Bell—motor and sensory nerves
1813	Davy on agricultural chemistry
1815	Chemical equations evolved
1819	Läennec's *On Mediate Auscultation*
1821	Steamships from Dover to Calais
1823	Stockton to Darlington railway
	Lancet started
1827	von Baer saw ovum
	Bright on renal disease
1828	Wöhler synthesized urea
1830	Lyell's *Principles of Geology*
1831	Chloroform discovered as a chemical substance
1833	Shaftesbury's Factory Act
	Müller's *Handbook of Human Physiology*
1835	Southwood Smith's *Philosophy of Health*
1838	Registration Act (births, marriages, deaths)
1841	Henle on microscopic anatomy
1842	Shaftesbury's Mines Act
1844	Wells uses gas in dentistry
1846	Morton and ether

	Telegraph Office in London
	Liston amputates with patient under ether anaesthesia
1847	Simpson experimenting with chloroform
1848	First Public Health Act
	Marx and Engels' Communist manifesto
1849	Addison on adrenals
1851	Helmholtz introduces ophthalmoscope
1852	Sims on vesicovaginal fistula
1853	Queen Victoria accepts chloroform in childbirth
1854	Snow breaks Broad Street pump
1858	Virchow's *Cellular Pathology*
	Medical Act founds General Medical Council
	Pasteur proves no spontaneous generation of life
1859	Darwin's *Origin of the Species*
1861	Semmelweiss and puerperal fever
1863	Helmholtz and hearing
1864	Lister used carbolic spray
1865	Spencer Wells on diseases of ovaries
1869	Mendeleev's periodic table
1870	Education Act—primary education for all
1873	Clerk Maxwell's formulation of electromagnetic theory
1876	Koch's *The Aetiology of Anthrax*
1877	Manson finds filaria
1879	Pasteur grows streptococci from case of puerperal fever
	Manson and mosquitoes as disease vectors
1881	Pasteur and anthrax vaccination in sheep
1882	Koch on tuberculosis
	Wireless communication
	Takali prevents beri-beri by diet
1885	Corning introduces lumbar puncture
1886	Krafft-Ebing's *Psychopathia Sexualis*
	Hertz and electromagnetic waves
1890	Halsted and surgical gloves
1892	Ivanow and tobacco mosaic virus
1893	His and the cardiac conducting system
1894	Einthoven and electrical activity of heart
1895	Röntgen discovers X-rays
1896	Becquerel and radium
	Riva-Rocci's sphygmomanometer
	Babinski's plantar reflex
1897	Pavlov's conditioned reflexes
	Havelock Ellis on the psychology of sex
1898	Curies obtain radium from pitchblende
1900	Wertheim's operation for cancer of the uterine cervix
	Planck's quantum theory
	Mendel's paper on genetics discovered
	Freud on dreams
	Bordet and Gengou demonstrate antibodies
1901	Landsteiner's blood groups
	Wireless transmission to Newfoundland
1902	Treves operated on Edward VII for appendicitis
	Bayliss and Starling on hormones
	Carrel and tissue transplantation
	Midwives' Act
1903	Almroth Wright on opsonins
	Wright brothers fly
1905	Einstein's Special Relativity Theory
1906	Sherrington's *Integrative Action of the Nervous System*
	Wassermann reaction for syphilis
	Blair-Bell on pitocin
	Gowland Hopkins on vitamins

1908	Donald–Fothergill operation for uterovaginal prolapse
	Hitschmann and Adler on physiology of endometrium
1909	Dale on endocrinology
	Kocher on thyroid
1910	Ehrlich introduces salvarsan to treat syphilis
	Flexner produces poliomyelitis experimentally
1911	Flexner Report on medical education
	Medical Research Council
	Biochemical Society of London
1912	Crystallography
1913	Rutherford–Bohr atom
	Haldane on high-altitude physiology
	American College of Surgeons
1914	Kendall and thyroxine
1915	Carrel–Dakin irrigation of wounds
	Tetanus prophylaxis
1916	Einstein's General Theory of Relativity
	Gaskell names involuntary nervous system
1918	Starling's 'law of the heart'
	Holmes on gunshot wounds of the cerebellum
1919	Rutherford split the atom
	Alcock and Brown flew across Atlantic
1920	Medical Research Council
1921	Banting and insulin
	Marie Stopes and birth control
1922	Public radio broadcasting began
	Nobel prize awarded for biochemistry of muscular action
1923	Health Organization of League of Nations
1924	Electron spin described
	Einthoven's Nobel Prize for electrocardiography
1926	Baird and television
	Minot and Murphy on liver for pernicious anaemia
	Busch's electron microscope
	Harrison synthesizes thyroxine
	Collip and parathyroid hormone
1927	Heisenberg's uncertainty principle in quantum physics
	von Jauregg's Nobel Prize for treating syphilis by malaria
1928	Aschheim and Zondek's hormonal test for early pregnancy
	Prediction of neutrino by Pauli
1929	Fleming and penicillin
	Talking pictures
	Dale and Dudley demonstrate chemical transmission of nerve impulse
	Forssman's cardiac catheter
	Eijkmann and Hopkins' Nobel Prize for vitamins
1930	Landsteiner's Nobel Prize for blood groups
1932	Chadwick and neutrons
	Adrian and Sherrington's Nobel Prize for nerve impulse
1933	Morgan's Nobel Prize for chromosomes
1935	Domagk and sulphanilamide
	Joliot-Curie's Nobel Prize for induction of radioactivity
	Watson-Watt and radar
	Spemann's Nobel Prize for organizer in embryonic development
1936	Colebrook and Kenny use prontosil in puerperal fever
	Public television broadcasting
1937	Ruzcha's electron microscope
1938	Joliot and nuclear fission
	Florey and Chain working on antibiotics
	Dodds and synthetic oestrogen
	Heymans' Nobel Prize for cardiac control mechanisms
1940	Landsteiner and Wiener on rhesus factor
1941	Gregg on rubella and congenital abnormality

	Cournand and McMichael on cardiac catheterization
1942	Beveridge Report
1944	Schatz, Bugie and Waksman on streptomycin
	Butler's Education Act
1945	Atomic bombs used on Japan
1946	Nuclear magnetic resonance
1947	Nobel Prizes for sugar metabolism (Cori and Cori; Houssay)
1948	Start of National Health Service in UK
1949	Kurzrock and Lieb on prostaglandins
1950	Nobel Prize for work on adrenal glands (Hench, Kendall, Reichstein)
1952	Nobel Prize for paper partition chromatography (Synge and Martin)
1953	Krebs' Nobel Prize for citric acid cycle
	Lipmann's Nobel Prize for coenzyme A
1954	Nobel Prize for cultivation of polio virus (Enders, Weller, Robbins)
1957	Nobel Prize for synthetic curare (Bovet)
1958	Communications satellite
	Nobel Prize for genetic recombination (Beadle, Tatum, Lederburg)
1960	Richards and nuclear magnetic resonance
	Maiman and laser beam
	Nobel Prize for transplant antigens (Burnet, Medawar)
1961	Gagarin in Russian Vostok
	Christ Church Conference on graduate medical education
	Human Tissues Act
1962	Nobel Prize for genetic code (Crick, Watson, Wilkins)
1963	Starzl's first human liver transplant
1966	Nobel Prize for cancer (Huggins, Rous)
1967	Royal Charter for College of General Practitioners
1968	Royal Commission on Medical Education
1969	Neil Armstrong on the moon
	Nobel Prize for work on viruses (Delbrück, Hershey, Luria)
1970	Steptoe and Edwards on *in-vitro* fertilization in humans
1971	Sutherland's Nobel Prize for the action of hormones
1972	Nobel Prize for structure of antibodies (Edelman, Porter)
1973	Nobel Prize for animal behaviour (Erisch, Lorenz, Tinbergen)

Name index

It is impossible to categorize in one word each person in the following list. The description chosen has been that which seems best to fit for the purposes of this book.

Abernethy, John	1764–1831	Surgeon.
Adams, Robert	1791–1875	Physician, heart.
Addison, Thomas	1793–1860	Physician. Adrenal glands.
Adler, Alfred	1870–1937	Psychiatrist.
Adrian, Edgar	1889–1977	Physiologist.
Aesculapius		God of healing
Albinus, Bernhard Siegfried	1697–1770	Anatomist, surgeon, physician.
Albucasis	936–1013	Physician.
Allen, Edgar	1892–1943	Endocrinologist.
Allen, Willard Myron	1904–	Endocrinologist.
Anthony	fl.c. 300	Saint.
Apollo		Greek god.
Aquinas, Thomas	1224–1274	Saint.
Aristotle	384–324 BC	Physician, philosopher.
Arkwright, Richard	1732–1796	Engineer, water frame.
Aschoff, Karl Albert	1866–1942	Pathologist.
Asclepiades	fl.124 BC	Physician.
Auenbrugger, Leopold	1722–1809	Viennese Physician. Percussion.
Austen, Jane	1775–1817	Novelist.
Avenzoar	1072–1162	Physician.
Averroes	1126–1198	Physician.
Avicenna	980–1037	Physician.
Avogadro, Amedeo	1776–1856	Chemist.
Babinski, Joseph François	1857–1922	Neurologist.
Bacon, Francis	1561–1626	Philosopher.
Bacon, Roger	1220–1292	Franciscan friar.
Becquerel, Henri	1852–1909	Physicist. Radioactivity.
Baer, Carl Ernst von	1792–1876	Embryologist.
Baillou, Guillaume de	1538–1616	Physician.
Baillie, Matthew	1761–1823	Pathologist.
Ballantyne, John William	1861–1923	Obstetrician.
Banting, Frederick	1891–1941	Physiologist.
Barclay, John	1758–1826	Anatomist.
Barnard, Christiaan	1922–	Cardiac surgeon.
Barr, Murray Llewellyn	1908–	Cytologist.

Subject index

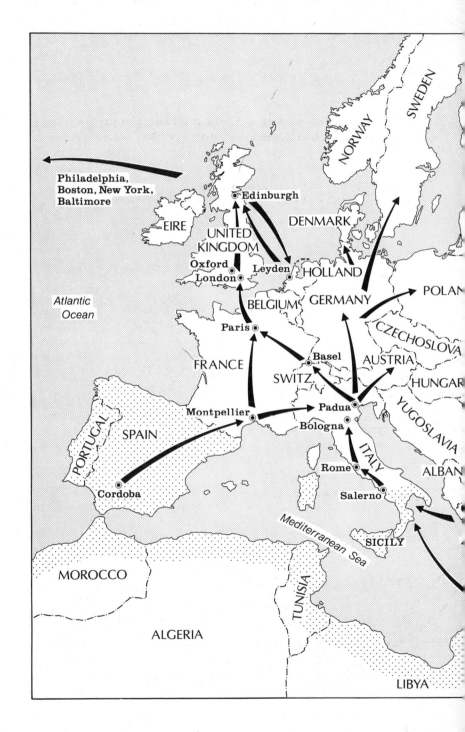

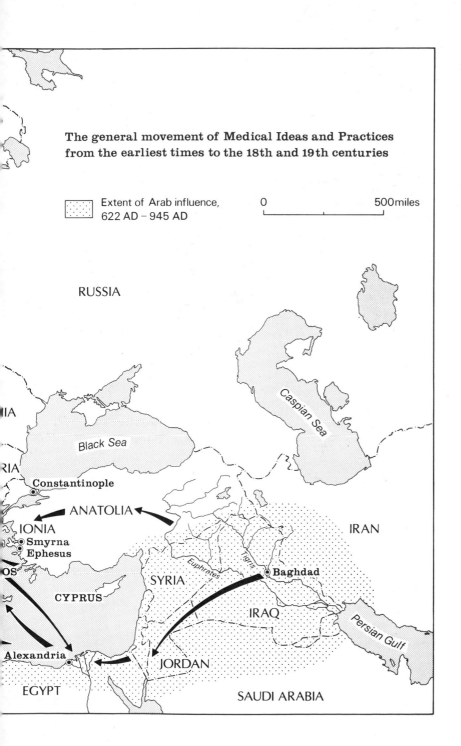

The general movement of Medical Ideas and Practices from the earliest times to the 18th and 19th centuries

Extent of Arab influence, 622 AD – 945 AD

0   500 miles

RUSSIA

Caspian Sea

IA

Black Sea

RIA

Constantinople

ANATOLIA

IONIA

Smyrna

Ephesus

IRAN

OS

Euphrates

Tigris

Baghdad

SYRIA

CYPRUS

IRAQ

Persian Gulf

Alexandria

JORDAN

EGYPT

SAUDI ARABIA